Love Start

Pre-Birth Bonding

Love Start

Pre-Birth Bonding

Eve Marnie, R.N.

 HAY HOUSE, INC.
Santa Monica, CA

Hay House, Inc.
501 Santa Monica Blvd.
Santa Monica, CA 90401

First Printing, June 1989

10 9 8 7 6 5 4 3 2 1

The author of this book does not dispense medical advice or prescribe the use of any technique as a form of treatment for medical problems without the advice of a physician, either directly or indirectly. The intent of the author is only to offer information of a general nature to help you cooperate with your doctor in your mutual quest for health. In the event you use any of the information in this book for yourself, you are prescribing for yourself, which is your constitutional right, but the author and the publisher assume no responsibility for your actions.

Certain names in *LoveStart, Pre-Birth Bonding* have been changed to protect the privacy of individuals who very kindly shared their stories in the hope of benefiting others.

ISBN 0-937611-38-7

Library of Congress Catalog Card No. 88-82325
1. Childbirth   2. Prenatal Care   3. Parenting

Text Design: Kevin Allen Pike
Text Photos: Daniel Ishmael Olmos

Typesetting: Highpoint Type & Graphics, Inc., Claremont, CA
Printed and bound in the United States of America by Delta Lithograph Co. of Valencia, CA

Dedication

This book is dedicated to
Nicholas Marshall Walsh and to
Neal and Kelly Marshall Walsh
whose energy and drive led to the
creation of this book.

Table of Contents

Foreword

David B. Chamberlain, Ph.D.
Author of *Babies Remember Birth*

Eve Marnie has written a passionate book introducing pregnant mothers and fathers to the joy of communicating with their unborn babies. She has been a cheerful pioneer on this new frontier of prenatal bonding and, I predict, her enthusiasm will be catching.

I am glad to have played a part in her quest for scientific validation of what babies can sense, learn, and remember before they are born. This has been my quest, too, since 1975 when I was suddenly confronted with lucid adult memories of birth. For me, that discovery led to a new world of knowledge about babies and their consciousness.

The idea of talking to babies in the womb is unusual but not exactly new. For centuries—perhaps from the beginning—mothers have done it, some shyly, some boldly, without being able to justify the practice. One of my clients, having a womb memory, described her mother's behavior this way: "Sometimes she talks to herself, but she is really talking to me. She feels silly talking to me so she is talking to herself. But she is really talking to *me*." Today we would say this mother was following her intuition.

Parents who want a *scientific* basis for relating to

their unborn babies can surely find it now. Indeed, they are in step with the times, heirs to an unprecedented breakthrough of knowledge about the unborn and the newborn. But this is a new development. You will still hear disclaimers from experts not yet familiar with the scientific basis for prenatal bonding or its psychological importance.

Only thirty years ago medical texts were saying that newborns were virtually blind, their hearing dull, and their brains nearly useless. With this poor equipment they were not expected to use their senses, express emotion, or have any awareness of how they were being treated. It was heretical to suggest that they could learn, remember, or be traumatized at birth.

In those days the placenta connecting mother and baby was considered a "barrier" protecting the prenate from the real world outside. Malnutrition in pregnancy was said to "spare the brain." These wishful ideas fit the general assumption that the period between conception and birth did not count. Parenthood would start at some later time. Now we know how false that was. Alcohol intake at the time of conception carries a specific risk of producing facial abnormalities, and the greater the intake the higher the risk. Malnutrition results in brains of lower-than-normal weight, length, and size. All parts of the shrunken brain suffer: neurons, synapses, neurotransmitters, and myelin sheathing.

Embodiment proceeds at a brisk pace. We know, by the week and day, just when and how each part of the physical body is developing. Sensitivity to touch, clearly present at seven-and-a-half weeks after conception, progresses steadily so that by seventeen weeks nearly every part of the body responds to touch.

By just ten to twelve weeks after conception, coordination of body and brain is sufficient to permit an active program of physical exercise. These graceful, spontaneous movements, observed by sonography, involve all parts of the body in bursts of activity lasting as long as seven minutes with rest periods no longer than five minutes. The fetus is busy in there!

The special senses come on line gradually. The mechanisms for tasting are in place by fourteen weeks, which means that prenates are able to taste during the twenty-eight weeks before birth. Swallowing speeds up for sweet substances, and stops as soon as a bitter taste is detected in the amniotic fluid. What the mother is eating or drinking, the baby is eating and drinking. If a mother (or father) smokes, the baby suffers the toxic fallout. Drugs, prescribed or unprescribed, taken in adult doses also reach the baby in *adult* doses. The connection between mother and child is intimate and inescapable. Quality counts.

Especially important is the hearing connection. All hearing equipment is in place about halfway through pregnancy, making it possible for the fetus to tune *us* in. This is voice-link, a private family line. Sound conduction by bone and fluid brings in sounds of the mother's body and her immediate environment (music, stories), especially the pitch of her voice. Research with elaborate sound portraits (spectrograms) of an infant's cry about *halfway* through gestation has shown that the baby has already learned some of the speech characteristics of his mother by this time.

Building on this capacity for hearing, a Canadian father, whom you will read about later, established firm communication and played a nightly game of "tag" with his unborn child beginning in the twenty-fifth week after conception—fifteen weeks before birth. This demonstrates not only hearing but learning and readiness for friendly interactions long before birth. Science is indebted to individual parents for discoveries of this magnitude.

Evidence of infant intelligence is easier to gather *outside* the womb, of course, and can begin to be found by studying babies born prematurely. These babies show us what was previously hidden from sight, the last ten or more weeks of development. Surprisingly, babies born ten weeks early have been found to be dreaming almost 100 percent of the time they are asleep. This makes them the biggest dreamers on earth. From every measurement, they dream like we do. Good dreams cause them to smile, bad dreams cause them to squirm and writhe. Their facial expressions are appropriate and adult-like.

By forty weeks, the usual time for birth, your baby will have all his senses. Tasting, smelling, and hearing are about as good as they ever will be. Vision is far advanced including color perception, a degree of depth perception, and even the rudiments of eye-hand coordination. The ability to adjust focus over a wide range (for example, from microfilm to freeway signs) will take a few more months to perfect, but at birth your baby will be able to see you perfectly well. When that gaze is turned on you, you know that a person is looking at you.

Parents soon discover the intelligence behind an infant's cries. Cries are compelling and persuasive signals, yet none are alike. Different cries reflect different needs and different circumstances. Experts once proclaimed that infant cries were "random noise" and meaningless, just as they said smiling was "gas," and pain reactions were only a "reflex." Actually, all of these are part of an impressive communications repertoire which exists long before birth. We are only beginning to acknowledge that babies—born and unborn—speak universal languages: cries, smiles, hand gestures, body movements, facial expressions, emotional outbursts, reactions to pain, music, color, flavor, odor, and voices. Babies are more ready to communicate with *us* than we are to communicate with them.

LoveStart is an invitation to early parenthood. The

steps Eve Marnie has outlined begin with the simplest interactions of resting, enjoying, and sharing with the person who is being embodied in the womb. As you follow this path, your personal bond with your child growing, you will surely avoid one of the tragedies of our time: reluctant and indifferent parenthood resulting so often in poorly constructed baby bodies that are born too soon and thrust into forbidding incubators.

The steps of *LoveStart* will bring you to the momentous decisions facing parents today about *how* to prepare for birth, *where* to give birth, and *who* to invite to assist you. In the age of medical birth, when these decisions have become so complex, this book will be a trustworthy guide for you and your baby.

Introduction

So much emotion, planning, and expectation attend the birth of a baby. We mark the event with a giant mental signpost: "New life starts here!"

In the meantime, we observe the growing signs of pregnancy and continue to do the same things that we have always done, until that dramatic moment when the new arrival forces us to take our habits by the scruff and simply toss them out.

New evidence mounts each year about the abilities of babies to hear, taste, see, feel, respond, and to remember the months of life before they are born. My professional and personal experience with childbirth, and realizing that my own children apparently received information in the womb, compelled me to write this book. For years, I have been working with expectant mothers and fathers as a nurse and as an instructor of birth preparation classes. The essence of what I have learned and taught is that the relationship—the love—between the parents and this new person must begin before birth.

LoveStart is an art, a science, a philosophy, about becoming acquainted with an unborn child through a process called PRE-BIRTH BONDING. Acquaintance, always a gradual process, results in friendship and begets a meaningful relationship that serves a lifetime. We first notice some feelings of fondness, move a little closer with each moment, and eventually, to our delight and surprise, we discover love. Becoming acquainted with a baby in the womb is a gradual process, not an abrupt event. It starts with the sounds, tastes, feelings, and movements a baby experiences before birth. Bonding includes knowing just what your baby is up to as he* develops.

The technical foundation of this book involves studies in the area of fetal development, the emotional transference called *imprinting*, and the metaphysical definition of the beginning of life. Discoveries in these areas will, in all likelihood, astound you as much as they did me. We have just begun to explore the back of that filing cabinet called *memory*. Parents are advised: "Your baby is 'listening in'. Your baby will remember!" The unborn child starts learning and relating to you long before birth.

We are about to explore the evidence for birth memory and its exciting implications. We will look at the ways an unborn child communicates to us, and how we can communicate back. We will share methods to make these pre-birth experiences pleasant and loving, and to make the grand event of birth itself less traumatic.

I believe this book will help you, your family, and its future generations grow, and have wonderful and loving first memories.

I am a nurse, so I suppose I could have been far better prepared for giving birth. Yet, at the birth of my first child, in 1972, when they clamped my wrists in restrainers, a feeling of cold rage and total helplessness

---

* The unborn baby, naturally, can be male or female. For editorial consistency, we generally refer to the baby as "he."

swept through my body. The spinal injection was one thing, quite bad enough, thank you, but physical immobilization was something else altogether.

My husband could see my frustration and despair as he stood just a few feet from me. I knew that he, too, was angry. But he had promised me earlier not to make a fuss on my behalf, and he was being true to his word, though I could see him working hard to restrain himself.

I had first found out about the use of wrist clamps and spinal injections at a Red Cross class I attended shortly after I began a childbirth preparation class. I remember seeing these techniques in a movie. I was horrified. "Not me," I muttered to myself. "They'll never do that to me."

You must understand that nurse or no nurse, this kind of approach to the beautiful and breathtaking process of birthing was totally foreign to me, in the literal sense of the word. In New Zealand, my homeland, no such methods are used. There, through all my nursing experience, I had never seen anything like it. My eyes popped out when I saw that Red Cross movie. The next day, I ran to my American nursing colleagues at a San Diego hospital.

"They do not really use those things, do they?" I asked. It seemed incredible to me that as a working nurse in this facility (although not in the delivery unit), I had no idea what was going on around me.

"Oh, sure they do," my friends confirmed. "It is standard procedure." I repeated the oath I had made to myself at the childbirth class. "Not me," I said. "That will never happen to me."

But it did happen. And it happened so fast, under the circumstances of labor, that I was unable to do anything about it, at least not without making a major scene right then and there, something I was in no mood to do.

Now, I ought to say that all this is not a major catastrophe. Every year, thousands of women give birth this same way. Indeed, across America, this way seems medically preferred.

I wanted to play a more active, a more here-and-now role in the birth of my child. I wanted to feel the wonder of giving new life. I wanted to hold my baby, touch my baby, establish loving contact from the very first moment. The "medically-preferred process" allowed me to do none of that.

My daughter, Marnie Bowen, was born shortly after 7:00 a.m. on July 26, 1972. I had labored through the night, but it was not a difficult labor at all. The doctors and nurses, I remember, were surprised by how comfortable I was. I had made the decision to use a natural childbirth method months prior to her birth. It was serving me well now. My husband stayed at my side, lovingly assisting, encouraging, and just being there for us; for all three of us.

Everything was going as I had anticipated, as I had always wished. Then, as dawn approached and I began to feel a little more discomfort, a tall, handsome, strange man approached me. My doctor, the man with whom I had formed a special partnership over the many months for this special moment, was nowhere in sight when Marnie chose to make her entrance. Another member of the corporation we now call "the doctor's office" came in his stead. I realized then that I had made a mistake. I could have asked to meet all the members of the "firm," so that at least I would have a passing acquaintance with whomever might ultimately assist me in the delivery of my baby. (I now advise everyone who uses one of the modern medical corporations to do this.) It never occurred to me (at the time) that my own personal doctor would not be there with me at the appointed hour. How naive I was.

"Would you like some medication?" the tall, dark

stranger asked me. I was unnerved by the sudden appearance of this "interloper" at my bedside at such a vulnerable time (although I realize now, of course, that he was a perfectly nice man simply doing his job). I was unnerved, too, by his question. Did he not know I was using natural childbirth? Had he not at least spoken to my doctor about my plans for this occasion? Had my special partnership with my physician, forged through the pregnancy, been in vain?

I, of course, had no way to measure things, no basis on which to take stock of how things were going. This was, after all, my first experience. Will the discomfort get worse? Will it turn into real pain? Will the moments ahead be excruciating? I asked the expected question.

"What do you think, doctor?"

"Well," he replied in a voice very kind and reassuring, "have a little something."

So I had a little something, meaning, a painkilling drug given by injection into a muscle.

I became a little sleepy, a little drowsy between contractions, but I could still feel things. I was comfortable. That was not such a bad compromise, I thought.

Through my drowsiness, I found myself next in the delivery room. It was time. Marnie was on her way. All the waiting, all the loving, all the emotion already invested. This was it!

The doctor sat me up on the delivery table, but he was not lying me back down. I felt a chilly, damp swab at my lower back. "Oh, my God," I thought. "An injection. They are preparing me for an injection!" My mind raced through the corridors of the sedation, trying to power through the gentle veil which that earlier "little something" placed between my thoughts and my actions. The words seemed to take forever to get to my lips. "Do not . . . I do not want . . . do not do that . . . ."

My husband told me the words never got to my tongue. He never heard them. He only saw the words all over my face. Before an actual sound was uttered, I felt the tiny prick of the needle at my spine, the urgent pressure of the fluid going in.

"Too late," I said to myself. Score one for the system.

I was too drowsy, only too much wanting to lie down to care anymore. A post-protest would accomplish nothing anyway, I reasoned, except to make every medical person in the room suspicious that because I was a nurse, I was going to be trouble. (Medical people hate to treat other medical people who always think they know best, and who start barking and ordering as if they were in charge instead of in bed.)

In the midst of this mental process of acceptance, I felt my wrists being clamped. My husband took a step forward, a quick, jerking motion. His face filled with questions. Is this what I wanted? Had I said something to them during one of the few moments he was away from my bed, being scrubbed down so that he could enter these hallowed portals? Would he break his promise? Would he make a fuss?

If he was looking for an answer, he got no help from me. My mind was too fuzzy, my eyes showed no sign of anger, only darting to the left and right, looking at my wrists now in restrainers. I caught his glance, but could send him no signal. I was in their hands now. The process of birthing was going to be their way.

The baby was almost out, anyway. She had begun to crown—that is the top of the baby's head showing— even before they had me on the table, which was another reason I wanted so desperately to lie down. Sitting there on the edge, getting the injection, I thought I might crush the little head by my own weight. Why would they have me *sitting* like this? I remember thinking, "I can feel the baby *under* me!"

Now all properly injected and clamped, I surrendered my will to the team of professionals around me.

How many times, I wondered, had my patients surrendered in just this same way to me? And how many times had I, in my role as God-of-the-Moment, failed to fully inquire about their wishes?

Marnie was being born now, and I felt nothing of her arrival. Oh, a little bit of pressure, perhaps. A little sensation of movement. But nothing of the real feeling of her arrival.

Then she was here. The doctor placed her on my stomach for one brief (very brief) moment. I looked at her, but I could not touch. I so wanted to reach out and touch. I wanted to hold. I wanted to embrace. I wanted to caress. I wanted to say with my hands what my eyes could not say. "Hello. Welcome. I love you. I am your mother. These are the hands that will always keep you safe."

The natural movement of my hands to Marnie was interrupted by the restrainers. "I cannot, I cannot hold my baby," I thought. Her own tiny arms searched the air for mine. She was crying, of course, and so was I.

They wrapped her up and took her away from me, after only a few seconds. They took her away! She was handed to my husband, who carried her to another part of the room that I could not see. And then she was gone.

I lay my head back down and stared at the ceiling. This was it. And now, it was over. I did not feel anything of the birth, and I could not even touch my child after she arrived. It was over.

Four hours later, after the recovery stage, they brought her to me. Only then was I able to establish physical contact with Marnie.

I recalled that fact nine years later, in the summer of 1981, when Marnie came to me with a puzzled look on her face.

"Mommy," she asked. "How come you never hold me?"

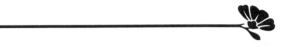

Discovery

It is a fact of my life that my oldest daughter, Marnie Bowen, gets held every bit as much as her younger sister, Barbara. Perhaps even a trifle more. She was my firstborn, and there is always that unique bond. Yet, Marnie carries an experience of not being held.

I dealt with Marnie's question as best I could at the time, reaching out and holding her right there on the spot, of course. I assured her that I had held her plenty of times in the past and would do so many times in the future. I never received the impression that she was completely satisfied with that, but both of us got through the moment.

For my part, I pondered for days. Where could she have picked up on the lack of being held? How could such a thought be true for her? I searched and reviewed my memory bank. I examined all of my previous behaviors. "No," I said to myself. "It is not true for me. It is not my experience." I had treated Marnie with every bit as much love, every bit as much physical contact as Barbara. With respect to touches and hugs, there was absolutely no difference between the two.

Then a thought struck me. "No," my left brain said to my right brain. "No," my logic said to my intuition. "That is preposterous. Ridiculous. And it has nothing to do with it." But my right brain intuition would not stop. It kept sending me contrasting pictures of Marnie's and Barbara's births.

Things were different at Barbara's birth; I had made certain of that. There were no spinals, and there were no clamps. When Barbara arrived, I reached out and held her, touched her, the moment she was born.

"That is the difference," my right brain allowed. And then my left brain logic took over. "Could that be the difference?" And could a child of nine years carry memories of her first moments so vividly as to bring the impression of these moments forward as a "life truth?" Is there such a thing as a *birth imprint*?

Marnie's question in 1981, and our shared experience at the time of her birth nearly a decade before, began the long search which has culminated in my life's work and in writing this book. For that question has led to another, even more startling inquiry: Is it possible that imprinting begins even before actual birth?

All living animals know things innately. A cursory scrutiny of animal behavior will make this clear. Babies know things innately, too. But where does this knowledge come from? How can a baby, long before he could possibly acquire sufficient data to render value judgments, make them?

When my second child, Barbara, was a newborn, she stubbornly refused to take milk from a bottle. From anyone. And it was not simply formula to which she objected. She not-so-politely declined expressed breast milk, too. For Barbara, it was mother or nothing.

Other babies took bottled milk. Why not mine? It was not a question of trying the bottle and then deciding she did not like it. She would not even try it. How could an infant show such a preference? On what basis had she made her very apparent decision?

During the early stages of my pregnancy with Barbara I made some firm value judgments. My baby, I determined, would be breast-fed. Later on, I decided that feeding my milk to Barbara from a bottle would be acceptable on those rare occasions when I would be away at feeding times, but this somewhat more practical decision was made after Barbara's birth. Is it possible she had been already imprinted with the original, less complete data? Could it be that such pre-birth decisions and feelings of the mother actually have a cognitive impact on the child in utero? When the child is born, does it know something because it was taught during gestation? Where does instinct come from?

Does the lion cub know things out of the experience of its mother before its birth? And if this is so, have we been ignoring that perhaps the most important time to educate our offspring is while the children are in utero?

These are the thoughts that filled my head in the late summer-early fall, 1981. I began watching both Marnie and Barbara for other signs of birth imprinting and pre-birth imprinting. I mentally logged the behavior of babies with whom I came in contact, as well. I saw films, read books, and drew some conclusions.

Babies are born with ideas. Lots of them. They know what they want. It is not babies who misread parents. Infants are reading us loud and clear. Even before a baby begins to see things clearly, that baby has a very good idea of what is going on.

The power of the mind's eye was demonstrated when I went for my first visit to a chiropractor's office. He worked with me, handled me, treated me for an hour, and walked me out to the desk to pay the bill. Only on my second visit did I discover that he was blind. Though I learned he had only recently lost his vision, I still marveled at how he could work so smoothly, so efficiently. "But, you do not see with your eyes," he said to me. "You see with your mind."

His words hit me like a brick. I began watching my own behavior, and all of life, more closely. I saw that my dog *knew* if he was in danger of getting a spanking or a hug, no matter how I approached him. One day I heard someone say, "That looks like a nice person." I have felt the same way about people, based on some intangible thing I picked up with my mind, not my eyes.

If babies are picking up *their* knowledge in the same way, who can say that this process begins only after birth?

"No one!" my right brain intuition shouted as I explored this question. I knew my intuition was right, that the baby is sitting there, like a computer, recording every piece of information he receives before, as well as after, birth.

I knew this was true. I felt it deep inside. But I wanted to have it confirmed. I felt a need to find a source outside of myself to confirm and agree. Isn't it strange how we can absolutely know something in our heart and still need external confirmation?

I suspected babies could hear in utero. I had been working out in an exercise class and two of the instructors were pregnant. They taught the aerobic exercises all the way through their pregnancy. These same instructors came to the exercise classes after delivery, putting their babies to sleep lying on the floor with heavy rock 'n' roll music blaring overhead. I stared at these babies, saying to myself, "This is not right. Babies do not sleep in this kind of noise." As I continued to stare at these sleeping babies my mind was screaming, "They could hear in utero. They could hear! These babies are used to this music. It is familiar to them, hence, they can sleep to it."

These days, I listen to what my intuition tells me much more closely. But at the time I had these thoughts, I had not yet learned to trust. "Good grief," I said to myself, "I am going to have to research all this. I have got to find out if all of this is true!"

"But how," I asked myself, "am I going to do it? It could take years."

The answer came as soon as I asked the question. And it came, in part, through the person who had started me thinking about all of this in the first place: Marnie.

I had been discussing this whole question with several of my friends, including my daughter. Marnie is very bright for her age. She understood my curiosity about these things. She rather enjoyed the idea of my working to solve this mystery of how babies come to know things, or come to have certain impressions of the world which they carry into later life.

One day, upon my return home, she said that a friend had called on the telephone. "She told me to tell you there was this TV show today, all about how babies understand things! Even before they were born!"

"Oh?" I said. I searched the TV schedules and discovered that the program must have been: "Out of the Mouths of Babes." It had aired on our local Public Broadcasting station. I set the information aside, making a note to myself to try to watch a repeat of the show.

A week later, on a morning after my husband and I had spent an evening away from home, Marnie came to me again. "There was another one, Mommy," she said. "There was another show about babies on TV!"

She remembered the show was "In Search Of ...Life Before Birth." It starred one of her favorites, Leonard Nimoy.

"This is too much!" I said to myself. "I have got to find out what this is all about!"

I called the television stations, both the one showing the Nimoy program and the local PBS station, and through some questioning, discovered that both programs included the pioneering work of psychologist David B. Chamberlain. I could not believe that he lived in San Diego! And when I checked the phone book, I nearly fell out of my chair. His office was just a few blocks from me!

Dr. David Chamberlain was the source I had been looking for. I contacted him immediately. He listened to my theories and concepts and invited me to his office, where he shared with me his then unpublished manuscript of a work he had been putting together, after years of research. The title sang to me, *Babies Remember Birth.*[1]

I hurriedly flipped open the manuscript, scanning the pages as fast as my eyes would carry me. It did not take me long to get the thrust of Chamberlain's message.

"My God," I said. "It appears you have documented what I believe. Babies are listening, learning, and remembering from the womb!"

Realization

I was born in Auckland, New Zealand, in 1939. At age fifteen, immediately after graduating from high school, I developed a strong interest in nursing while working in a doctor's office. As the doctor's only employee, I worked as a receptionist and also with patients in the examining room.

Following this job, I worked in the laboratory at Auckland Hospital, on the North Island. At eighteen, I went to general nursing school at Christchurch Hospital, where I stayed on as a staff nurse when I graduated at age twenty-one.

In a year, I became what is known as a "sister" (this is not related to any religious order), which is similar to a position as head nurse in other countries. It was unheard of for a person of my age to hold such a post.

In my mid-twenties I began to cultivate an interest in teaching, yet I wanted to find a way that I could teach and still be with my patients—not be stuck in some classroom or lecture hall somewhere. I went to Melbourne, Australia when I was twenty-five to accept a position at the Royal Women's Hospital. I took a one-year training in midwifery and won a gold medal for Best Practical Midwife.

Then I went to the Australian outback where I was a bush nurse doing deliveries; after that, I went on to London, England, to work as a private duty nurse in a hospital intensive care unit. There I was named head floor nurse.

By thirty, I was married and living in the United States, where I completed requirements for Registered Nurses' certification. I have been working as a staff nurse at Mercy Hospital in San Diego since 1970 where my background was recognized by the hospital administrators, who asked me to teach childbirth classes. I have been teaching them most Wednesday evenings ever since.

That is my background in brief. I have always had a tremendous interest in the subject of childbirth and a variety of prior experiences from which to explore the subject.

After talking with Dr. Chamberlain, and reviewing his startling research, I naturally began to ask myself new questions. What can I do with this information? How can I help people to use it?

The door that Marnie opened for me when she questioned me in 1981, and the door through which I walked to meet Dr. Chamberlain, placed me in a state of awareness, a state of receptivity for new information, new clues that would confirm, or add to, my intuitive perceptions about both birth and pre-birth imprinting.

I know that birth imprinting is nothing new. The concept has been discussed and explored before, by scholars, doctors, psychologists, and laypeople. The subject of *pre-birth imprinting* is another matter. Not much has been said about this possibility in either medical or philosophical/psychological circles.

I would like to play a part in changing that, because I believe the topic is so important, so vital to the future of our children, and hence, to the future of the planet.

You might ask, is this not a bit of an overstatement? Have we not gotten along quite well without it for these many centuries? The answer is all around us. No, we have not! We are fighting wars which need not be fought, building personal frustrations which need not be built, holding fears and guilts which need not be held. We are sending people to mental institutions who need not be sent, taking tranquilizers and drugs which need not be taken, experiencing uncounted moments of personal pain, sadness, and anxiety.

In short, ours might be a healthier world, a happier world, and a more loving world, if we look to our own beginnings, and the beginnings of our children, to launch the next generation in a different way.

This I firmly believe.

If you ask me for proof of these concepts and theories, I would ask you only to look at something new and surprising: *birth memories*. Perhaps the one person who has done the most to bring these before the public is Dr. David B. Chamberlain. He has recorded hundreds of birth and womb memories since 1975, including the one, taken under hypnosis, which follows:

Dana Remembers Her Birth

Labor and Delivery:

Dana: I seemed to be insecure; I didn't want to come out. Some kind of pulling and tightening. Movement, lots of movement; myself moving.

Dr: You didn't want to come out?

Dana:	Didn't. No. Safe inside; didn't want to come out. A lot of noise. Lots and lots of noise, and just confusion outside.
Dr:	Do you know where you are and who's around?
Dana:	I'm in an operating room, or some kind of hospital room. A lot of chrome instruments. A metal table. And my mother's on the table. And there's a lot of men and women—seven or eight—dressed up in gowns. They're all talking and rushing around. My mother's in a gown, white-blue gown.
Dr:	Are you already out or still inside?
Dana:	I'm still inside, but it seems I can see the room right now; I can see where it is, and there's noise and confusion. My mother's really, really nervous, but she's not all there, seems like. She doesn't seem awake or have her eyes open. Her eyes are down, shut. I can't see anything else.
Dr:	Can you follow the conversation, notice what they are concerned about?
Dana:	No . . . I can't get the words.
Dr:	Come forward to the time of labor and delivery.
Dana:	I'm being squeezed. My head is being squeezed and pushed down. A really small area; a real small area. Really, really squeezed. I'm going down a canal, and I'm trying to get out. I'm moving slowly, slowly; not very fast. I'm coming out slow, and it

seems I'm being moved by the skin surrounding my head and my body. And I'm coming out.

And then there's light, lots of light. Really bright. Really bright. And it seems like something's on my head or by my head; seems like I'm just being pulled out by someone or something. There's one big bright light in particular. I'm being pulled out and very scared; very scared!

Dr: How much of you is out?

Dana: Just up to my waist. And I'm out. I'm out! As I'm being pulled out I'm rushed up, yanked up by the feet; one leg first, then the other. The blood's rushing to my head; it's very uncomfortable. They're slapping me, really hard, on my rear end; bottom of my back and my rear end; and it hurts.

Then they do some suctioning with some kind of tube in my nose and mouth. And I'm handed to a nurse after my umbilical cord is cut, which is really quick. Everything was so quick! It wasn't done slowly and softly. It was done quick and rushing-like.

Dr: Did it bother you when the cord was cut?

Dana: There wasn't any pain; it was just a security gone. All of a sudden I wasn't connected . . . I'm scared and I'm upset and I'm crying; really crying out loud. And then my mother's saying, "Oh God, it's a girl! It's a girl!" The doctors—it seems like there are two men—are holding the baby, and then the nurses take me away. I'm angry!

Dr: What about?

Dana: How they treat you. I wasn't held gently; I was grabbed at. It was a rush thing—wham, bam, spanked! Then picked up and grabbed and shown to my mother, who wasn't all there . . . She didn't get up. She just laid there . . . Her eyes were closed for a minute and then she noticed me. A lot of people were talking. Everybody's talking at the same time. And then the nurses take me away.

Separation in the Nursery:

Dana: I'm going to another room. I just see the hallways and I feel very, very, very scared. Two nurses walked down the hall with me, and it was very bright. Very bright. My eyes were hurting and I was crying. Then I was brought to another room where I was cleaned up and (they) put a diaper on. It seemed very rushed. Very pushed around. Rushed. Put my diaper on, and everyone had masks on.

Then they put me in the incubator and closed the lid. I'm put in a white room in a glass box and there are other babies around me. I'm on a white, soft pad, but I'm feeling so frightened and upset! I'm crying. And one of the nurses said to the other, "What a pretty baby!" I'm lying on my back, my legs moving and my hands are scratching my eyes, scratching my eyes and nose. I'm crying, screaming, and I'm getting out of breath.

Dr: Do you know what you're frightened about?

Dana: There's nothing surrounding me, nothing holding me. Too much open space! Too much freedom for my arms and legs. Air; too much air. Not too much *air*, too much freedom . . . I'm not curled up safe.

Dr: It's not what you've been used to.

Dana: No, it's very different, very different. And it's also very bright. Too much light. It hurts my eyes. My eyes are stinging, really stinging. There's tears coming out of my eyes. The blood feels like it's rushing toward my head, my shoulders, my chest. Very hot. I bumped my hand against the glass. It's just so different!

Dr: Different from being inside, you mean?

Dana: Yes, very different. It's dark and safe inside. Nothing's comfortable (now).

Dr: How long does this last?

Dana: It seems like hours . . . Women come in and look at us, touch us. Cold hands; really cold hands touching us, and with masks on, covering their nose and mouth. And everybody's crying. All I can see is me in the incubator.

Dr: Is it just a bed or is it an incubator?

Dana: It's an incubator. It's small and it has a lid on the top. It has a white pad, a white sheet. I didn't have anything on but a white diaper.

Dr: How long were you in there?

Dana: Hours. Hours. Hours—I don't know how many hours . . . A lot of hours, it seems like.

Dr: How did you like being in there?

Dana: I didn't like it. I didn't like it. I wanted to be where I was, inside my mother. I just didn't feel very secure. No one to hold me, tell me everything's okay . . . Oh God! It was *so* upsetting . . . (whimpering, then crying). I needed her to hold me. They should have let her hold me. I wanted to crawl back inside again.

Reunion with Mother:

Dana: She's holding me, and I'm in a blanket, a white blanket. She's looking at me, touching me. She's smelling me! (chuckling) She's smelling my breath. She's smelling my breath and my skin. She asked the nurse why my toes were so funny. She thought they looked funny all curled up. The nurse said that's just the way my toes are, that they weren't deformed; she was concerned about that.

I felt safe in her arms, warm. I felt better not closed in a box. I felt safer. She was nervous how to hold me. She didn't know if she was holding me right. She seemed uneasy, but excited and happy . . . She kept changing sides to hold me.

Dr: What kind of place are you in?

Dana: I'm in a hospital room with a bed, and there's a nurse in there, and somebody else . . . I feel so much relief. I see mother in the hospital bed with propped up pillows and she's sitting there feeding me (a bottle). It doesn't taste that good; it tastes like vitamins . . . I'm sleeping (now), very quiet. Sleeping. Comfortable.

Dr. Chamberlain's Comments:

Dana's birth report is typical of the many I have heard, but unusual in the fact that it was obtained under research conditions where the mother's report, also in hypnosis, was used as an objective measure of its reliability. It proved to be a report with no serious contradictions and nineteen points of correspondence with the report of her mother.

The young married woman giving this birth report is Dana, age eighteen. She had no conscious memories of her birth and had a mother who claimed she had never shared any details of the birth with her. She had never done any work in hypnosis before but adjusted quickly to it and completed her memories in about three hours. The segments of her full report given here are: labor and delivery, separation and nursery time, and reunion with her mother.

In hypnosis, thoughts come forward slowly, painstakingly, with great reflection. Words are carefully chosen and sometimes do not fall into formal sentences and paragraphs. The impression is one of engagement in awesome self-discovery, becoming reacquainted with deep inner knowledge or viewing some kind of record that is coming clear, moment by moment.

Adult reports come in adult vocabulary, of course, not baby talk. Vivid recall of the past does not mean regressing to the age involved. Nor do clients abandon their intelligence while having memories; the superior mental resources of the present are tapped. Consequently, a birth report is a report of birth put into the best language available. This is how people reporting birth can speak of things like vitamins, doctors, and incubators which were presumably not in their vocabulary at the time.

In cases where the birth setting has involved a different language from English, my clients have automatically translated their reports into English, with only passing quotation of key words in the original tongue. Regardless of the language in which a report is couched, it is a report of experience. Even if babies know nothing of doctors and nurses to begin with, they quickly discover how they act and know how they react to them.

Instant learning seems to take place. Thinking, and even intense efforts to communicate that thinking, is evident, though these efforts are not generally appreciated by the adults present. Occasionally, newborns are profoundly affected by specific words or sentences spoken to them at birth. They quote these verbatim and tell their reactions to them.

How these words can have such devastating and lasting impact when formal language does not develop until later, is something of a mystery. It helps to remember that formal language is only a vehicle for communication. Communication itself *is* mysterious. Sometimes it is wordless; telepathic. Children may be better at this than adults because they are not yet distracted by formalities of language. Communication flows from *action* (we see and understand) and from *emotion* (we feel and understand). We often "get the message" *before* it arrives in words.

When words have unusual importance, I believe they become engraved in our consciousness. My experience with hypnosis leads me to accept the reality of some deep level recording which keeps essential data intact. Indeed, without such a record, there would be no possibility of the kind of playback we encounter frequently in hypnotherapy. Those who have had near-death experiences sometimes report that they "saw" their entire life flash before them. A well-trained clairvoyant can "read" a person's history by "looking" at it, further evidence that there must be some kind of *record* held in the mind.

From a therapeutic point of view, these early memories are important because they can influence the way a person thinks, feels, and lives. We are not dealing here with grammatical abstractions waiting to become real at some future time. Memory is alive and dynamic. We act out our memories, tend to be programmed by them to be afraid or trust, to feel confident or anxious.

As is typical of all other reports of birth, Dana displays a keen perception operative *at the time*. She reports the differences between the inside world of the womb and the chaotic outside world. She says the adults at her birth are noisy, all talking at once, strangely out of touch with her presence and needs. She realizes that her mother is very nervous and drugged, "not all there." When the cord is cut, it is done in a rush, with no apparent awareness on the doctor's part that her *security* has been abruptly severed. She feels disconnected—a matter which seems to be of no concern to anyone else!

In the delivery room, all is haste. There is pulling, rushing, yanking, slapping, grabbing, revealing gross insensitivity. Lights hurt her eyes. They sting. Her little hands bump against glass. The nurse's hands are cold—a glaring environmental problem. There is crying, crying, and more crying—a sign of something wrong that no one seems to take seriously or read correctly. Events after birth are sterile and strange: "I was brought to another room where I was cleaned up . . . it seemed very rushed . . . put my diaper on, and everyone had masks on. They put me in the incubator and closed the lid. I'm put in a white room in a glass box . . ."

Her plaintive appeal from the nursery is typical: "No one to hold me, tell me everything's okay. Oh God! It was so upsetting. (Crying) I needed my mother to hold me. They should have let her hold me. I wanted to crawl back inside . . ."

🐚

This documentation of intelligent memory—and my discovery through Dr. Chamberlain that other researchers throughout the world were coming to the same conclusions—is what gave me the impetus and courage to move forward with my own plan. I wanted to deal with the implications of these findings in a practical way; to put what I already knew to be true to work for mothers and babies.

Consider the implications:

- *Consciousness* is well-developed at birth and begins long before.

- With an active mind before birth we are busy forming impressions of the environment and learning from all our experiences.

- With repeated impressions, we can become convinced about things, form definite patterns and beliefs.

- We may unconsciously live out these "truths" for decades afterward unless damaging imprints are altered.

- The education of our children proceeds at a brisk pace at birth, so we have reason to be more careful about *what* we are teaching them. And what might they be learning *before* birth?

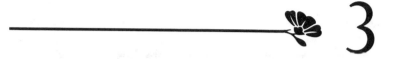

3

Truths

These are the truths I want to shout to the world: that newborn babies can *hear*; that babies can *see*; that babies can *feel* emotions (yours and their own); that babies can think and comprehend and decide. And if babies can do these things, how might the expectant mother and father influence the baby who is still in the womb?

If mother and father have a big argument, is baby not affected? If mother and father share a loving, tender moment, does baby not pick up the vibes? If mother and father are scared, or worried, or joyous or depressed, the baby receives these messages about the world into which he is soon to be born.

Yes, the messages received by the child, the impressions formed, the "truths" accepted, depend to an extraordinary extent upon the messages, impressions, and truths the mother and father send him.

Just as one would not scream and fight and throw things and create a frightening scene in front of an infant, one must also not do these things in the presence of the soon-to-be-born.

Another pioneering researcher in birth memory is Dr. David Cheek, an obstetrician in San Francisco.

Dr. Cheek kept meticulous records of births. Years later when using hypnotic regression with adult patients, he found they could demonstrate the exact head and shoulder movements involved in their own births. This was confirmation of body knowledge, cellular memory, or imprinting carried in memory from birth.

Evidence for this kind of memory was also brought to public attention by psychologist Arthur Janov in his books *Imprints* and *The Primal Scream*.[2] Dr. Janov was the originator of primal therapy, a type of therapy that brings out intrauterine and birth memories. Often, secret information, such as the method of an attempted abortion, is revealed in this therapy. Think how it would startle you to have your grown child tell you of such events you thought were known only to you.

In *Mind-Body Therapy*,[3] Ernest Rossi and Dr. David Cheek discuss the idea of cellular memory. They note that one does not necessarily need a fully developed brain to remember; body chemicals carry messages. In the baby's brain, some of these chemicals are found as early as six or seven weeks into the pregnancy. Found throughout the body and in electrical circuits of the brain, the chemicals carry information back and forth. According to Rossi and Cheek, messages from parent to baby can be remembered, especially the highly charged emotional ones. These messages can become *imprinted*.

Imprinting is a relatively new term for the transference of feeling from one person to another.

In his paper on imprinting at birth, Dr. Cheek defines imprinting as any emotional response that becomes fixed by the emotional or physiological stress with which it first appears.

Imprinting, according to the Random House Dictionary, is a rapid learning that occurs during a brief receptive period, typically soon after birth, and establishes a long-lasting behavioral response to a specific individual or object as attachment to parent, offspring, or site.

So, if babies are truly aware of what is going on at the moment of birth, when does this awareness begin? When the child is one inch out of the mother's body? Halfway out? With the first breath?

Clearly, for a child to have picked up impressions of his own birth, conscious thoughts have to be taken in by the mind from a period before birth.

This raises tantalizing questions. When before birth? How far back into the pregnancy? How soon following conception? This leads to the age-old question of philosophers and theologians: When, exactly, does life begin?

My own answer came to me intuitively.

"If what you say is true," my questioner began, "if what you theorize has validity, you must have an idea as to when this pre-birth process all starts."

Without thinking for so much as a moment, I said, "I do. It begins as soon as life begins. Not life outside the womb, but life inside the womb."

"And when is that?" my questioner wanted to know.

"Why, I suppose it would be when the heart starts beating," I replied. "It is rather logical, isn't it? If we accept the fact that life—at least, life as we know it and define it on this conscious earthly level—ends when the heart stops beating, does it not make sense to assume that it begins when the heart starts?"

The name of my organization formed in support of this message was "born" at that moment: HeartStart-LoveStart. Yes, of course! That's what it is all about!

Prior to this flash of understanding, I was not opposed to abortion. The statements above, which are true for me now, naturally threw my ideas and thoughts on abortion into turmoil. If what I have come to understand about the beginning of life is *true* (and I repeat, for me it is), then could I condone mid-term or late-term abortion?

The answer is not simple. Abortion is an uncom-

fortable subject. Every time I speak out in public, the
question is raised about abortion. Each of us has to
make our own decision about the issues. I believe each
woman makes the decision that is best for her, given the
circumstances, her moral beliefs, her individual beliefs,
and the best information she has at that moment. If you
had an abortion twenty-five years ago, or yesterday, you
made that decision with the best knowledge you had.
Today we have more scientific information to consider.
Still, you may wish to proceed with an abortion in the
future, knowing full well that the pre-born baby experiences the event. But there is another side to the issue of
abortion: the pre-born baby's point of view. How do you
know that, metaphysically speaking, the baby does not
choose to experience the event? What is the difference
between choosing to live or die at twenty-five years or
at a few days or weeks after conception?

So, proceed with caution as you rush to instruct a
woman about the rights or wrongs of abortion, for the
moral issues are endless and we are only beginning to
take a metaphysical look at this complicated issue. If
you have had an abortion or are contemplating one,
remember the spirit or mind of this person you are part-
ing from, or have left. You still have grieving to do or
some process of uncoupling or separating to consider.
Realize this person may have chosen to leave.

I often wonder about the Sudden Infant Death
Syndrome. Does the baby think, "Oh, I made a mistake!" and leave? We seem to require a medical reason,
and we need to consider spiritual purposes, as well, as
they apply to our lives. Since I do not wish to turn this
book into an argument for or against abortion, that is
all I am going to say on this subject. I wish this book
to deal primarily with how we can produce happy,
healthy, loving, joyful, wonderful people out of the
experience of pregnancy and birth. That is what this
book is about.

Many parents do not even start loving their baby until months after the child's birth. It is sad and true that in some households, one or both of the parents do not begin relating to the child until he at least begins to act intelligent, to crawl, to walk, to talk.

In the minds of some parents, there seems to be a difference between an infant and a baby. An infant needs constant care and attention, morning to night, and does very little but eat, sleep, cry, eliminate waste, and grow. The infant becomes the baby later on down the line.

It is tragic that in some cases, for this reason, many children do not receive the love and attention they deserve as living, breathing human beings until late in the game. There are parents who do not even relate to their child until he uses all his faculties. This is because of the gross misunderstanding in the minds of many parents as to just what the baby comprehends. If parents think that until a baby crawls, walks, or talks that the child is not functioning mentally on a very sophisticated level, they will say things, for instance, that they wouldn't say in front of an eight-year-old. The child, they reason, does not understand anyway.

Arguments will take place, worries will be expressed, depressions will be acted out, all manners of behavior will be displayed in the home of newborn infants as if there were only two people living in the home, only two people whose feelings need to be considered.

In this way, many babies are treated on a level only slightly higher than pets. Their presence is noted, they are cared for, their basic needs are served, but they are truly seen and not heard, and they are seldom considered at all on a level which acknowledges their own thoughts and emotions. It is assumed they have no thoughts or emotions.

Those people on the cutting edge of scientific

research and philosophical exploration in this area are providing us with thought-provoking information. Babies not only have thoughts, feelings, emotions, and consciousness as infants, they also have these faculties before they are born. And these feelings, thoughts, and emotions are in no way limited to the pre-born's experiences *inside* the womb. Conditions, conversations, circumstances, and events occurring outside the womb can also affect the baby.

Ask any mother who has carried a child for nine months. Why does the baby sometimes start kicking when mother is upset? Does mother's emotional state truly create a response inside the child? You bet it does.

Babies are astute at determining mothers' emotions. Intrauterine bonding is a fact of life. Mothers describe it and babies demonstrate it. Perhaps being aware of her baby's feelings may assist a pregnant mother to make emotional adjustments of a positive, loving nature.

We might describe the baby's experiences with us as "bonding" emotionally. Joseph Chilton Pearce, author of *Magical Child*,[4] describes bonding as furnishing points of similarity between what has already been learned and the new. The joy of looking at this word *bonding*, with its implication of *becoming acquainted with*, is to pause and perceive that this may be the way all learning is acquired.

Bonding works both ways between parents and unborn babies. The parents become acquainted with the baby, the baby with them. On the physical level, rhythms of life are also a part of bonding. Sleeping patterns established in the pregnancy continue after birth. In his book, *The Birth of a Father*,[5] Martin Greenberg, M.D., calls bonding "engrossment," a delightful term that describes a father falling in love with his newborn baby. Engrossment is something wonderful to look forward to!

Another tribute to fathers and their empathy with

women comes from Dr. Jack Heinowitz in *Pregnant Fathers*.[6] Bonding is demonstrated very beautifully by men who, with incredible empathy, gain weight and suffer morning sickness and sleepless nights during their wives' pregnancies! Dr. Heinowitz separated groups of expectant couples, with men in one room and women in another, asking the same symptomatic questions of both groups. Surprisingly, often the answers were identical! We might pause and acknowledge men who show such unconscious sympathy and who are attuned to their wives and children.

If babies remember, see, hear, feel, and relate to us while they are in the womb, then this is *pre-birth bonding*. Because this may be when the deepest impressions are made, I have developed a program of pre-birth bonding, which lays out for parents a "curriculum" to make contact with the child. Since a bond is made with the child whether or not we want it, the question is, of what nature and quality will that contact be?

The bonding process can begin immediately after parents discover the pregnancy. After the *communication phase* (steps one through five) comes the second half of pre-birth bonding, the *action phase* (steps six through ten). Parents can follow this basic outline:

1. Rest

2. Enjoy the Baby

3. Make Contact with the Baby

4. Begin Conversation

5. Share Your Whole Life

6. Visualize

7. Educate Yourself

8. Prepare for the Birth

9. Put Your Plan into Action

10. Experience the Birth

The fifth step, share your whole life, continues after baby is born and throughout the child's life. I impress on new parents the importance of changing life patterns. Among other things, this helps the parents identify with the child. Then, when the baby arrives, he does not feel like a stranger in the home. A child's feelings of being an interloper are eliminated if the mindset of the parents is altered even before the baby's first heartbeat. When the first beat is struck, the baby senses a welcoming, accepting atmosphere. He knows that he has been expected and has been loved, even in advance of his physical arrival.

Who among us does not feel wonderful when we arrive at the home of another for a long-awaited visit and find ourselves greeted with the words, "Come in! We have been expecting you! We couldn't wait for you to get here?" How many babies are greeted with these words and emotions? How many are greeted with these words and emotions even before they are born?

So, let us look more closely now at pre-birth bonding. Let us examine how you create a loving, welcoming space for your family's newest member.

❧

The first step in pre-birth bonding is: REST.

It is an important first step, and yet many expectant mothers do not undertake it until relatively late in their pregnancy. Unless there is a rash of morning sickness or an early onset of physical fatigue associated with

the pregnancy, some mothers have been known to continue life as usual, including their often hectic schedules, until their physical condition forces them to slow
down.

Setting aside a rest period each day is the first step
in pre-birth bonding because it sets up a routine. This
will be very important later on. This time is set aside
not only for the mother's physical health, but to let the
baby know that this time is for him each day.

The baby comes to know that he is important, and
has become, from the very outset, a part of your daily
life. Resting involves not only the mother, but the
father, too.

Each day both parents find a time when they can
be together with the child. This will be a restful and
peaceful period. Parents, do not sit down in front of the
television, or have a quiet dinner together and say:
"Well, that is our quiet time with the baby for today."
I suggest setting aside a time each day that is exclusively
for the baby. This may be as little as ten minutes in the
early stage of pregnancy. The time will lengthen as
there is more to do with the child.

At first it may feel strange to sit down, or lie down,
together for this "quiet time" with your child. There
will seem to be nothing to do. I start the pre-birth bonding process with resting to get you used to spending this
exclusive time with your child, to give you a chance to
push through your own initial feelings of strangeness
and awkwardness about this daily event, to get you to
accept this time as normal and natural, good for both
you and your child.

Later, when you actually start talking to your baby,
it will seem much more natural to do so if the *three* of
you have first learned to spend some quiet time
together, simply recognizing and acknowledging each
other's presence.

Like tuning up a car before a big trip, the first step

in pre-birth bonding tunes the body and the mind for what is to follow. It sets up a routine and establishes a procedure. It gives both partners an opportunity to move to a place of appreciation and understanding of the event that is changing their lives.

A good time for this initial rest period is in the morning just after awakening, or just before going to sleep at night. You are in a rest mode anyway, and the time spent this way will seem much less awkward.

I suggest that mother and father simply lie together quietly for a few minutes. You may hold hands or just cuddle. You may wish to center your thoughts on the baby who is on the way; to think about what your baby will look like and what you want the baby's life to look like as well. The mental planning can begin now. I do not suggest talking at this stage, although there is certainly nothing to prohibit it. It is just that talking tends to lead to daily considerations and sometimes moves the process away from your child. So, until your mind is trained to allow this time to be focused exclusively on the baby, I find it works best for these few minutes each day to be observed in silent togetherness.

Afterward, when the ten or fifteen minute period is up, you may wish to share your experience about this time; what came up for you; what thoughts and ideas and images you created; what concerns arose in your consciousness and so forth.

Mainly, the rest period's purpose is to establish a daily routine. It is a way of saying, "This is the time we will spend each day in the bonding process, getting ready to welcome our baby." Like exercising, it is important to move into the bonding process early, slowly, and deliberately.

Many parents find other benefits from this first step. Believe it or not, many couples go months, if not years, without spending so much as fifteen minutes together in conscious silence. Many parents, having once established this rest period routine, continue it long after their baby is born. They would not miss it for the world. For a while, they proceeded with the rest period routine as an effort to begin bonding with the child, but they soon discovered that it also led to a re-bonding of their own partnership. Quiet time together, without a word being spoken, but with a conscious holding of each other in thought and emotion, will have a tremendous impact upon relationships.

This is not to be confused with silent times together while driving long distances, or while one reads the paper and the other does the dishes. I am talking here of quiet time in which each embraces the other in consciousness and each embraces the coming baby as well.

Unborn babies are conscious, wonderful persons in utero, deeply involved in becoming acquainted with their world and ours; dependent totally on the parents for a loving, nurturing, and cherishing environment. The question to consider is: What would your baby prefer to experience in utero? As you integrate pre-birth bonding into your life, consider your baby and the messages your baby receives about all the aspects of your lives.

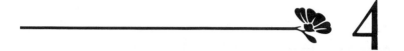

4

Joys

After the first step, a daily rest period, is established, pre-birth bonding moves to step two: ENJOY THE BABY.

Adults know that it is one thing to be with another person and still be alone in a space—be it a room, a car, a house, or whatever. It is quite different to be in the same space and know that someone else is consciously sharing the moment with you. So, too, is it quite different for the unborn child to experience relative isolation in the womb and then feel some other living being with him. Make no mistake about it, the baby knows the difference. That is the whole point of pre-birth bonding. Enjoy the baby by thinking about and conversing with him.

While thinking of your baby, you may begin to quietly share the excitement about the new arrival, your plans and dreams, ideas for baby's room, baby's name and baby's clothes, and even long-range hopes for your baby's life.

Enjoy your child. Enjoy the fact that the child is coming. Enjoy the future by imagining it. Enjoy running through the many names and the many possibilities for the baby's life. Share the glory of what has occurred in your family life. Use these few minutes together to get accustomed to talking actively each day about what is now going on in your life. If the pregnancy has come as a surprise, if there is any reluctance or hesitation about having the baby or about what changes the baby's arrival will produce in your family's life, use this time to talk lovingly and openly about it. Square away feelings and come to an understanding about how things will be. Be honest. Share openly. Do this each day.

By no means must enjoying the baby be limited to these few minutes each day. Yet, it is important to routinely set aside these precious moments for just that purpose. I can assure you that the process will reap untold additional benefits. Just as many married couples spend astonishingly little time together in conscious silence, a remarkable number of couples have never gotten into the habit of setting aside a few moments every day to simply talk together, to talk about what is going on with them, what their concerns, hopes, dreams, and directions are for the next day to the next week or month or year. These things seem to come up once in a long while, only after arguments, after a quiet evening together, or when something unique or damaging happens in their lives.

I know many couples, for instance, who never talk about money until the big and usually unexpected expense comes along. Then, in the midst of the crisis, they begin to communicate about the whole subject of finances. The same is often true in other areas of mutual interest and the same may very well be true of the baby's arrival.

I have been discussing the impact the pregnancy will have on you, while saying little about the impact it will have on the unborn child. Yet this is the main reason I have developed pre-birth bonding techniques. Babies know, feel, and intuit that they are being thought of, spoken of, loved, and consciously included in the lives of their parents. That is why parents who virtually ignore direct communication with the child until after he is born are doing a disservice to both themselves and the child. Have you ever watched your dog lying silently across the room, seemingly oblivious to what is going on? Have you ever noticed that as soon as you start thinking about the dog, its tail mysteriously starts thumping against the floor even before its eyes are open?

This is a common phenomenon. Feelings, which are manifestations of thoughts, travel across space and through barriers. Babies in the womb react to feelings. It is as simple as that. Feelings travel distances that words often do not traverse. Feelings, even more than words, are mental, emotional outputs. They are received in the deepest part of us. They are received and perceived, intuitively, often even without words being spoken. Go to a party and look across the room. Observe two people in conversation. Notice how you cannot at all understand the words being spoken, but can easily pick up the feelings being exchanged between the two. Remember the times you have caught the eyes of your loved one across a room. Remember the times, when in these instances, not a word was spoken. Remember how easy it was to receive feelings. A child of two years can perfectly understand feeling. A child of one can do the same. So, too, can a child of one week. There is no question about this.

Pick up an infant and love him. Just look at a child with love and watch the response. Have you ever thought of a far-off friend or loved one, then suddenly received a letter or a phone call from that person? Have you ever laughed at this apparent coincidence and said, "Oh, I was just thinking about you!" Can this be a coincidence at all? Thoughts and feelings are products of individual universal intelligence. They are received by universal intelligence as well. Think lovingly of a plant every day and watch it grow! Think lovingly of inanimate objects for that matter, and watch for a response! Absurd? Crazy?

How many times have you attempted to start the car in the morning to no avail, then patted the dashboard lovingly and said, "C'mon baby," and have it start right up! Write it off as nonsense if you wish. People reacting and interacting with the universe discover life itself reflecting their thoughts and feelings about everything. The baby inside the mother's womb is as much a part of the universe as anything else. A divine intelligence created this incredibly intricate form of life. Can it be possible that having done so, it left this living, growing baby incapable of receiving, understanding, and responding to the rest of his environment?

So, I assert that baby can understand the messages we send, perhaps not on the exact level we are so used to in our daily life, but most certainly on some deep intuitive level, the same level that makes plants grow, cars start, and people know what is being felt across crowded rooms.

I consider thought as very real energy. Often we seem to draw thoughts in at the same time. Some designs and products have been patented or produced at the same time around the world. For something to happen, an electrical energy and thought has to precede it. Henry Ford *thought*, then proceeded to invent the combustion engine. Thought is the most significant part of our lives. As a parent, be selective about what you are thinking. Thought seems not only to have electrical energy but also chemical energy. You may not believe your baby can pick up on your thoughts, but your baby is washed in chemicals that result from your thoughts and activities.

The power of thought has been written about often. Norman Vincent Peale wrote *The Power of Positive*

Thinking[7] and *Positive Imaging*.[8] In Ernest Holmes' and Willis Kinnear's Science of Mind book, *A New Design for Living*,[9] Plato is quoted: "If the head and body are to be in good condition, then we must first heal the mind and soul." Within recent years, the medical profession has confirmed that the mind-body connection is no longer theoretical. During the 1980s, much has been written about thought and its connection to disease. Paul Pearsall, in *Superimmunity*,[10] advocates the power of thought and its affect on our bodies. Dr. Bernie S. Siegel, in *Love, Medicine and Miracles*,[11] discusses how people he calls "exceptional patients," changed their thoughts about themselves and subsequently changed the course of their diseases—even cancer was cured. The most important thoughts seem to be about forgiving ourselves and loving ourselves. These thoughts assist in healing the mind-soul. Frequently, people use such methods, along with appropriate medical treatment, to assist the body to heal.

When you as a parent choose to place positive, loving thoughts around your baby, you create more love for your baby. Each of us can only live in the moment, so our thoughts at this moment are significant. In *You Can Heal Your Life*,[12] Louise L. Hay, metaphysical counselor, writes that you are in control of your thoughts. You choose them.

So, having established a routine of setting aside ten or fifteen minutes each day, as a couple, to contemplate the arrival of the baby, you can use this period to actively communicate about your life together as a family. You can expand your daily period of time together by adding on fifteen minutes or so at the end of your quiet time to share what you are thinking and what you are feeling. In this way, each day the intimate time with the baby in the womb grows from ten minutes to twenty, or from fifteen minutes to thirty. Some parents have convinced themselves that their lives are so busy that they do not have thirty minutes to be intimate with the baby. Tragically, many parents have not found thirty minutes a day to be with their children long after the children are born and well into their teens. Setting up a routine in the way I have suggested can gear the parents towards more participation in their children's lives for many years to come.

❧

Step three in pre-birth bonding brings you to the most exciting part of the communication phase: MAKE CONTACT WITH YOUR BABY.

Steps one and two begin immediately after discovering the pregnancy, or as soon as you discover the pre-birth bonding process.

It is hard to imagine this tiny human being as having a personality. It may be difficult to believe that this tiny person is taking in mental images of his own, but it is true. You are not dealing solely with the physical body of this being, but also with that which makes this body, undeveloped and tiny as it may be, a living part of the universe. You are dealing with the stuff of which humans are made. Some call this energy. Some call it the force. Some call it the spirit or the mind or the thought or the soul. Whatever you call it, it is undeniably there. It is fully developed and ready for business. It is that thing which makes every thought possible. It is life itself. Think of this life as having a personality, for it does. It has one massive personality, expressed in a million ways. Life, the force, the spirit, the mind-soul, enters the body and leaves the body at certain times. That life is intelligent. It knows what it is doing. It could not arrange itself in such miraculous ways without having pre-birth memories. Something is driving the physical molecules, atoms, and tiniest bits of matter into connections and interactions which form what we call beings. It is this being that I am talking about. It is this being with whom you wish to make contact in the bonding process. It may help you to understand that you are not trying to establish contact with the tiny body now developing within you, but with the intelligence behind that which is developing.

Under hypnosis, this intelligence has told us of memories from before the birth of the physical body it has adopted. Indeed, it has told us of previous lives. People have revealed information under a trance that they could not possibly have known without having pre-birth memories. So, the question for all parents becomes: What do you want this intelligence to know about you? You want the baby to know that you care and that you love the being who has arrived in your life. This is what contacting and bonding are all about.

Contacting the baby consists of thinking to your baby. Start by consciously sending your thoughts to him. Recollections of birth remain into adulthood in the subconscious mind of every person. So, it is the spirit of the child, the spirit-mind of that new life growing within the mother, with whom you are communicating. You may be having a rough time with that word, *spirit*. But it is the spirit, the divine intelligence, the universal life force, the very essence of your child, with whom you are making contact. What else could it be when we speak of a being four to six weeks after conception? That is why thoughts are the most convenient, and at this point, probably the most comfortable mode of communication.

If you feel a bit awkward at first, when communicating thoughts to your child, stop trying and just let it happen. Think intuitively. Think naturally. Talk to your baby through your thoughts as you would talk to any being of intelligence. Relax. Listen to music. Make physical contact by resting your hand on your tummy. Touch, with a loving and caring touch.

Then simply think to your child, "Hello. We are glad you have arrived. We love that you are joining us here in our life. We have been excited ever since we found out you are arriving. Everyone we love is already expecting you! They have started to pick out things they want to give you. Boy, are you ever going to be loved. We've been thinking of names. Nicholas Brandon, if you are a boy; Arielle Dawn, if you are a girl. We hope you like our choices. The important thing for you to know is that we love you." Be honest with your baby. There is no point in not being honest. Children can tell every time when you are not being straight with them. They certainly can tell just as well while they are inside the womb as when they are out. You cannot fool your own mind and you cannot fool another part of the universal one-mind.

If you have some considerations about your baby, let those considerations be part of your communications. "Boy, you surprised us! We were not expecting you just yet. We had it all planned out that we'd have children a little later. We are a bit worried about how we are going to afford some of the expenses. We know that it is all going to work out. We love you, and love makes everything work. If we seem a bit worried now and then, just kind of go with that. We have not quite mastered not worrying yet!" Yes, you can use humor. Yes, you can communicate whatever is natural. You do not have to use baby talk either, anymore than you have to after the baby is born. Any thought you can think, your child can comprehend. There is no thought too sophisticated.

Now we come upon a difficult subject. What if your baby's arrival was not entirely a happy occasion? What if there is apprehension, concern, even anger? What then? Good. So much the better for you that you have decided to communicate about it, even if only in your thoughts. Say the truth in your thoughts. Let your thoughts always be what is true for you. Do not worry about the impact on your child. The child will understand. More important, there is a very good chance that, having thought your most nagging thoughts, you will be able to let go of them. Thoughts withheld are thoughts repressed or suppressed. Thoughts expressed are thoughts addressed. Very often, simply addressing an issue clears the air about it. This is true in adult conversation as well, although it sometimes can take us years to discover.

I once knew a man who swore he did not want a puppy in the house. Everyone else in the house wanted one, but he kept saying he did not want the bother or the trouble. The other family members prevailed when, as life would have it, the family's youngest came home one afternoon, puppy in tow. "He followed me home, Daddy!" the child exclaimed.

The father's immediate response was, "Well, he can just follow you right back out again!" But somehow the puppy stayed. He jumped from time to time on Daddy's lap. He wagged his tail and hopped and skipped all around the place. And once, when Daddy thought no one was looking, he was caught smiling at the dog and ruffling his wonderful, soft hair.

It was not long before apprehension turned to unconditional love. So, too, it is in nearly every case with children. Do not berate yourself, or feel guilty, if you do not feel completely comfortable or happy with the timing of your new arrival. Do not worry that you are worried. Do not berate yourself if you cannot find a way to feel totally happy over the present turn of events. Simply be honest about it with yourself, with your mate, and with the child.

And trust. Trust that where love is given and love is received, every condition is healed.

In step three, I also encourage the mother and father to use their previously established time together with their baby to commence touching. Father may lovingly touch, caress, and even gently massage mother's abdomen. Later in the pregnancy you will actually be able to feel the baby move and kick. Obviously, for father-to-be, it is more difficult to come to grips with the fact that the baby is actually in there, living and growing. It is one thing to understand something intellectually. It is quite another to gain firsthand knowledge. In many situations, the mother alone experiences the growth and development of the baby. The father may become involved only after the baby is born, or, in some cases, many months after. Many fathers do not begin to relate to the child until it crawls, walks, and talks.

Pre-birth bonding is a way to share pre-birth nurturing and growth, just as the experience of conception is shared. The period of pregnancy is not a father's nine innings on the bench. It is a precious time, a time of immutable truth and magic, a time when the union of mother, father, and child brings unspeakable rewards to all three. It is a time of beauty, delight, surprise, and love. It is a time that comes only once with each child and so a time to be treasured. It is a time to be tenderly shared.

You can create a time of loving touch, when the baby will come to expect that touch each day. Consider touching to include hugs. Most people enjoy a loving hug from a friend. Presume your baby would love to be massaged, touched, and hugged. Small children often hug pregnant bellies. Later, you can use this time of touching to look for and identify your baby's body parts. Explore, caress, and feel your growing child. Touching your baby in utero brings confidence in touching your baby after birth. Many fathers report that as a result of pre-birth bonding, they are confident with the baby afterward. They say, "I would have been looking through the nursery window, instead of being here holding my baby in my arms."

Touching your baby in utero brings response. Your baby may draw away, wake up, kick, or push toward you. You will enjoy the pleasure of becoming aware of your baby's movements and behavior. You will notice various rhythms of life, patterns that are consistent with your baby. You will notice individuality being expressed. Looking at touch from your baby's point of view, we find your baby becoming acquainted with his environment. Your baby is touching the walls of the uterus, touching the cord, and touching his own limbs and body. We know scientifically that your baby can pull away from a touch on his cheek at seven and one-half weeks into the pregnancy.

Touching and abdominal massage during the pregnancy leads to easily giving your new baby a massage. This will prove useful when your newborn is fretful. Familiar with your touch and knowing it represents love, your new baby can respond and settle down, provided the baby is not sick or hungry. Videos, tapes, and books are available on infant massage. In some cities, there are classes for new parents. Dr. Ruth Rice[13] of Dallas, Texas, has done much pioneering work in the field of massage for premature babies. Scientifically, it has been documented that newborns gain weight and generally do much better when they are touched and massaged, especially when it is done by the parents.

In *Touching*,[14] anthropologist Ashley Montagu writes that regular body caressing by the father is so important that it ought to be standard obstetrical practice. The touching and caressing commenced in early pregnancy ought to be carried into labor and delivery. Dr. Montagu reports that mothers who have been recently, appropriately, and meaningfully touched use their own hands more effectively with their baby. Skin contact promotes development of the newborn and simultaneously, it increases the loving and bonding. So you can stroke and love your baby in utero with loving abandon, continuing loving massages after birth, knowing you are promoting growth and development.

How to Have a Smarter Baby[15] by Susan Ludington-Hoe is a book written to enhance your baby's learning both in and out of the womb. Included is a system to stimulate and activate your baby's brain cells in the womb, using movement and touch.

In northern California, obstetrician Rene Van de Carr encourages the stroking and patting of the pregnant belly. At Dr. Van de Carr's "prenatal university," the baby is taught to associate certain sounds with certain movements. Contacting your baby opens up the worlds of thought and touch, which brings you closer to your growing baby.

Massage and touch are valuable for both you and your baby. One heart-warming story about touch comes from Candace Fields Whitridge, R.N., who practices midwifery with great joy, in the mountains of northern California. Whitridge outlines the unborn baby on the mothers' tummies to assist in pre-birth acquaintance during examinations. The mothers respond in various ways: faint interest, stroking the tiny fetus, giggling, laying baby clothes over her tummy to check the size of her baby. You can imagine the surprise when the pregnant mother comes home and pulls up her shirt to display a drawing of her expected baby. Whitridge's idea of pre-birth acquaintance and her intuitive skills help generate positive feelings in relationships where abuse and lack of communication exist.

Pre-birth bonding techniques cause the fetus to become more real to these parents and thus reduce the likelihood of abuse. I encourage you to ask your midwife or doctor to outline your baby on your tummy. Have fun with the results. At any time during the pregnancy, you and your partner can draw a picture of your baby. Attempt to draw the baby to the size and development you think it has reached at the time along in your pregnancy. Keep your drawings and family portraits in your baby book for later in your lives. Drawing your baby assists you in understanding his development. You can compare your drawings to drawings in Lennart Nilsson's book, *A Child is Born.*[16]

Another fascinating aspect of drawing is that you each draw the same baby differently! As you discuss these individual drawings, your individual attitudes emerge about the baby.

Judith M. Lumley, M.D., of the Queen Victoria Medical Center in Melbourne, Australia, published a paper titled "Attitudes to the Fetus Among Primigravidae."[17] (Primigravidae means the first pregnancy.) Dr. Lumley's study showed that many women, even medical professionals, had difficulty reproducing the size and growth of their babies in utero. I find because the videotape, *The Miracle of Life,*[18] is shown frequently on television and is available for rent, more couples than ever before are informed about the growth and development of their baby. In child development classes, an associate of mine, Dr. Mort Rieber, suggests you write a list of the strengths and characteristics you expect your baby to exhibit from each side of your family. These lists provide great discussions between couples.

In steps two and three, you are enjoying and contacting the baby. These joys continue to strengthen your relationship, for with love, joy, and sharing you are creating a special union with your baby. There will be no gift you can give your child to match it throughout his life.

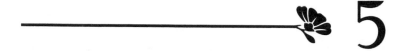

Sharing

Step four, BEGIN CONVERSATION, is an expansion of step three. Having established contact with the baby, begin talking to him. CONVERSATION leads into step five: SHARE YOUR WHOLE LIFE. It will seem like a one-way conversation for the first few months. During this time, it is worth remembering that appearances are deceiving. One-way conversation does not mean one-way communication. After the baby is born, talk to him soothingly and lovingly. Watch the smile cross his face. Is this smile not a return communication from your baby? You do not need the baby to say anything to know that your highest communication, the communication of your love and caring, has been received. This the baby gets. You can see the baby gets this because the message-receiving mechanism is right there in front of you. Yet, this message-receiving mechanism is not the baby. It is the baby's mind. If the mind is working while the baby exists in the womb, it is reasonable to assume your baby receives messages of love and caring in utero just as efficiently as he does following birth. But, is the baby's mind working before birth?

Biologically, there seems little doubt that the

brain, the physical tool of the mind, begins to function long before the baby is separated from the mother. It is clear that babies in utero hear, sense, feel, and react. Your baby is aware of his environment. More than one mother has been heard to say, rather proudly about the child she is carrying, "The baby seems to have a mind of his own today." Although the mother may not believe it, the statement is quite literally true. Babies kick and move, making it very clear when not enough nutrients are being supplied, when not enough rest has been received, and when insufficient attention is being paid to other emotional and physical conditions during pregnancy.

So, we know your baby's brain is functioning. The only question is, when does this begin? Generally speaking, biological death—that is, the end of the life of the brain—is associated with the end of the functioning of the heart. When the heart stops, life is said to be over. Brain waves have been known to continue briefly after cessation of heart activity. The two are closely aligned. So, it stands to reason then, that the brain may start when the heart starts. This is long before physical birth.

The brain probably responds to the environment around it both inside and outside the womb. If the first impressions are the most important and the most difficult to erase, all the more reason to surround your baby with soothing music, tender touch, and caring words. While the baby may not understand your specific words, I believe important feelings and meanings may indeed be computed and stored at some level of consciousness.

On a personal level, if someone you loved were in the same room with you, would you choose to not communicate with that person for nine months? Then, why do the same to your own child? Simply because your child has yet to be born is no reason not to communicate. I suggest that you begin talking with your child as soon as you are aware of the child's presence in the womb, for as surely as you are aware of your child, your child is aware of you.

Begin by creating a safe space. If you have followed the previous steps, such a space has already been created. Now, just add music, touch, and thinking. Then add verbal communication on your list of activities. This may seem awkward at first, but you can learn to do it.

I once saw an adorable three-year-old hug his mother's tummy and say to the baby inside, "Hurry up and get here!" Everyone thought it was cute, but the three-year-old seemed to be the only one in the room to whom it had not occurred that the words were wasted. Sometimes in life we find that to reap the richest rewards, it works to be as little children.

Approach the business of talking to your baby with the faith of a child. Tell your questioning mind to take a walk. Use your sense of intuition, your feelings of love, and your deep caring to make a bond with the baby. Your conversations with your baby can be about anything and everything. Simply say what you feel like saying. Talk about what is going on with you. Tell your baby stories, of your family's history, of your day's activities, of times you enjoyed and celebrated life. Introduce the world to your baby.

There is a wonderful musician, Andreas Vollenweider,[19] whose tape, "Behind the Gardens," has many different sounds, like laughter and a rain storm. It can be played in your home, and introduced to your baby. Reading or telling stories with music in the background is stimulating to both sides of your baby's brain. Voice tapes introduce other members of your immediate family to your baby, especially when they are far away from you. Grandparents can sing, play, or tell family history. They can read nursery stories or poems to your expected baby. Fathers who are frequently away may send voice tapes to play to the baby. The newborn child will certainly recognize the father's voice when the father arrives home. Read to your expected baby. Continue to read to your baby after the birth. A parent who reads creates a child who will enjoy reading.

Babies can hear from the womb. Mothers notice babies jump when car doors are slammed or react to loud noises such as airplanes overhead. Babies have been listening in for some considerable time during the pregnancy. Intrauterine sounds include blood moving in the mother's bloodstream, the mother's heartbeat, and the mother's voice. It appears we learn speech in utero. Babies born of mute parents either do not cry at all or cry with a very peculiar sound.

Apparently, a hearing baby can encode his mother's voice to such a degree that a baby born as early as twenty-two weeks has a voice print that can be matched to his mother's voice print. Psychologists W.S. Condon and L.W. Sander used high-tech cameras to photograph newborns listening to adult speech. They found that baby's movements were coordinated with the segments of adult speech. Evidence shows the baby is learning many life rhythms to the background of breathing, heart, and bloodstream sounds heard in utero. Professor James McKenna of the University of California, Irvine, School of Medicine, has written a paper[20] that describes how fetal breathing, fetal hearing, and fetal brain activity all develop at around the same time in utero, reminding the baby to breathe. Logically, these reminders continue after birth. McKenna explored the significance of fetal hearing and breathing in relationship to breathing after birth. We are the only mammals that give birth and then take the baby away from the mother. Is there some correlation between this and Sudden Infant Death Syndrome in our culture?

Understanding that babies can hear in the womb, parents may rapidly become acquainted with their unborn child when they play music—either a musical instrument they enjoy or a tape on a Walkman with the headphones placed on the lower uterine wall. Playing classical music, such as Vivaldi's "Four Seasons," which has a wide range of sound, stimulates the growth of more neurons in the brain cells. When you play music, the baby will respond.

How babies encode sound in utero is well documented. Dr. Anthony DeCasper[21] of the University of North Carolina has found that babies can discriminate sounds, and they show preferences for those which have been made familiar to them, particularly their mother's voices. Babies like familiar sounds.

In his book *The Secret Life of the Unborn Child*,[22] Canadian psychiatrist Thomas Verny tells the story of an orchestra conductor who found he could play certain pieces of music sight unseen. When he discussed the situation with his mother, a professional cellist, she said they were pieces of music that she had rehearsed over and over while she was pregnant with him.

Dr. Leon Thurman, co-author of "Heartsongs,"[23] an active guide to pre-birth and infant parenting through language and singing, is emphatic about the benefits of prenatal communication. Remember, many of you naturally sing to your unborn child and continue to sing to him after birth. For those of you who are hesitant because of your singing ability, "Heartsongs" will dissuade your fears about singing and relating to your infant. Dr. Thurman connects the growing teenage suicide and pregnancy rate to a lack of bonding between parents and their teenage children as babies.

Dr. Thurman, Dr. Thomas Verny, and Sandra Collier have researched the benefits of music in the pre-birth bonding process. They express some concern about babies hearing loud hissing noises at the end of a tape. You may want to record on a continuous loop tape, or obtain a music tape produced by Verny and Collier for the unborn child called "Love Chords."[24]

Keep in mind also, that your baby may like different

sounds than you do. A story indicating such a preference is revealed in the work of psychiatrist Rima E. Laibow[25] of New York. When her son was two and a half he commented on his birth and on the "window in the darkness." His very surprised parents asked him what else he remembered, as they realized, even though they did not believe it, that their child was telling them about his cesarean section birth. He also told them about the circular light overhead, the half-faces with green patches, being suctioned, and having something stuck up his anus. He remembered he felt cramped and painfully squeezed by the walls. Relating a personal preference during pregnancy, he said that the loud, low frequency notes sung by his mother were painful to him. Dr. Laibow had recalled that during the pregnancy when she sang certain low notes, her unborn responded in a very active way, but she had misinterpreted this as a happy response.

Using "Heartsongs" helps parents communicate with their babies. Through the use of language and music, cornerstones are being laid in the womb that will enhance your relationship with your child. When you are working hard, or are experiencing great pleasure, your body sends out chemical neurohormones called *endorphins*. So, under the influence of fun, pleasure, and song, your baby is washed in your endorphins as well as making his own endorphins—these are present in your baby as early as six weeks into the pregnancy.

Marc Freeman, Ph.D.,[26] of Queen University in Canada, writes about a husband and wife expecting their firstborn. The wife, using suggestions from Dr. Verny's *The Secret Life of the Unborn Child*, decided to read stories and sing to the unborn baby. The husband, not to be outdone, came home each day and pressed his face into his wife's tummy saying, "Hoo-Hoo!" At twenty-five weeks into the pregnancy, in response to the father's "Hoo-Hoo," the baby pushed on the abdominal wall into the father's cheek. When the father moved his face to the other side and said "Hoo-Hoo!" the bulge would follow. From that night on, they played fetal tag, and this continued for fifteen weeks before birth. In the delivery room, as the baby was breast-feeding, the father would make the "Hoo-Hoo" sound, to which the baby would stop nursing and search for the familiar sound.

Michel Odent,[27] obstetrician and author of several books on childbirth, uses music to prepare expectant mothers for childbirth. In France, where he made his observations on women in labor, Dr. Odent's childbirth techniques include discussing with expectant parents positions for birth, familiarizing them with the delivery area, and having them sing with his staff on a weekly basis. Imagine singing with your obstetrician! Dr. Odent feels there is a bond forged by song between the parents, baby, and staff when they sing together.

What a joy for you to experience your baby responding to the different sounds you introduce. Conversing with your baby leads to step five: SHARE YOUR WHOLE LIFE.

🐚

Sharing your whole life with the baby means just that. It is the crossover, too, from pre-birth to post-birth interaction. It means that after your baby is born, the special time which has been set aside each day to be with your child will continue.

Resolve to spend time with your baby. Play the same music and speak to the baby in the same way as before. Let your infant know that there is a unique time each day that is devoted to him. Continue this all during your child's life and you will notice a difference in the way your child relates to and reacts to the world.

The beauty of pre-birth bonding is that it establishes

a routine and builds a framework which makes setting aside a special time seem more practical. Parents often create the illusion that they are terribly busy and simply do not have time to spend with their children every day. Pre-birth bonding shows that a few minutes of direct and loving attention will add up to a lifetime of joy.

I do not mean setting up a routine whereby your child is addressed during a brief half-hour period each morning and then ignored for the rest of the day. Quite the contrary. The process will establish a link of communication, a bonding with the child which permeates the entire experience of child and parent.

You can send mental messages to the unborn baby at any time, for instance. "I am having a really rough day, and I am a little uptight right now, and you are not the cause of this. I am looking forward to your coming and I love you" can be an enormously comforting message for the child to receive on a day which is not going right for the mother.

Another subject to address concerning sharing your life with the baby is sex. Many parents-to-be feel uncomfortable about sex during pregnancy. The thought that your baby is actually registering the relationship of the parents can be mind-blowing. For most of us, the sexual experience is intensely private. The thought that your privacy is now interrupted by a third person may be difficult to handle. When most couples discuss their apprehensions about sex during pregnancy, they are usually referring to the physical aspects of sex. Some couples are afraid of hurting the fetus. In all but the most advanced stages of pregnancy, this is not usually the case, but you may want to check with your doctor.

Consider the message your baby may receive about sex. If sex is loving, gentle, warm, and wonderful, the baby will probably receive the mental message that the parents are loving each other in this perfectly natural and beautiful way. If there is resentment, anger, force, violence, or other negative behavior associated with the sexual experience, there may be an imprint on your baby's mind about sexuality. If you think any experience is inappropriate for your baby, you may want to make the appropriate change in your life.

Please note that impressions need not be permanent; they can be corrected. New messages along one line can wipe out or overpower messages along another. If you have an argument in front of your child as an infant or during the pregnancy, do not lash yourself with guilt; just notice that this has happened and move on. Resolve to bring such disagreements to a more peaceful settlement in the future. Decide to do better. Communicate more clearly and more quickly so that feelings will not rise to the boiling point. In this way, you change the messages you send to the child who may be observing from a crib or from inside the womb. If a sexual experience has been less than totally loving and caring, any message the baby has received because of it can be corrected.

The important thing is to have no apprehension, sexual or otherwise, about what is said and done during pregnancy. Live with love, understanding, patience, and kindness during this period, during all the days and weeks and months which follow, and your baby cannot help but get the messages you wish him to receive.

Sensitive obstetricians talk to preborn babies. A doctor I know talks to babies throughout the pregnancy and at delivery says, "You did a good job." He lets the newborn baby grasp his finger, and says, "I am sure you feel a little uncomfortable. Hold my finger until you are feeling better." This obstetrician is there for the baby!

Talking intelligently to your baby will prove useful and reassuring to your baby, especially in labor, when often you are concerned about the position of your baby for delivery. The baby may change position dramatically for you. This occurred to a couple whose baby was in a transverse lie (lying straight across the mother's tummy) one week before delivering. The doctor said a cesarean section would be the only choice. The father-to-be decided to talk to the baby about it. Placing his own head at the lower end of his wife's enormous tummy, twice daily, he whispered instructions to his unborn child. I do not know what he whispered, but sure enough, the baby's head moved downward, ready for normal delivery. The family believed, as I do, that the baby was curious and moved toward the father's voice. As a result this couple experienced a happy, natural delivery, when a few days earlier, they had been preparing for a birth by cesarean section.

In 1987, I was a labor coach to a close friend who was expecting twins. It was Linda's second pregnancy; she already had a four-year-old. She planned for a natural delivery. Linda was very small, weighing only ninety-four pounds prior to the pregnancy, and I suspected she would have a cesarean delivery. Linda commenced labor at 6:00 a.m. by breaking her water. She and I went to her doctor's office at 11:00 a.m. A sonogram showed the babies nose-to-nose under Linda's rib cage, and presenting their feet and buttocks for delivery. Her relaxed doctor sent her home to labor.

Linda labored intermittently all day with light, ineffective contractions, never settling into a proper, true labor. At 2:00 a.m., some twenty hours after her water broke, we were all tired. I suggested we prepare for sleep. I knelt down beside Linda and quietly discussed with the twins that we all needed sleep and that we needed to prepare for the cesarean section at 7:00 a.m. One hour later, Linda was in full labor. At 4:00 a.m., we arrived at the hospital and Linda was ready to push her twins out. During the delivery, I encouraged her with words of support about the great job she was doing. I talked to the twins during the birth process. I noticed the surprise on the faces of those in the room preparing for the sudden arrival of the twins. Linda's supportive doctor also talked to the twins throughout the labor. Shortly, we all proudly welcomed a boy and girl into our world.

Realize that you can remain with your baby even if the baby has to go to a special-care nursery. Babies do not like being alone. Adults regressed by hypnosis say, "We have been together for nine months. Why am I being left alone in a box now?" At some hospitals across the country, newborns are being examined by the pediatrician at the parent's bedside, rather than being taken away to a nursery. Explore this option.

Individual bonding by a parent is revealed in the following story. One woman reported to me that just after delivery, she heard her baby crying frantically in the delivery room and said to her husband, "Honey, do something!" Her husband, a truck driver, undaunted by the clinical nature of their hospital delivery room, stepped close to his child and sang a nursery song. The baby quieted and all was well. However, all was not well when the mother, a few days later, tried to quiet her crying baby with the same nursery song. The baby would have none of it. The song was connected to the father and would not work for the momentarily frustrated mother.

Frustration and stress are areas that often bring up fears about pre-birth bonding. If the baby can sense, can feel, can understand by his intuition what is going on in the environment, then what about the times when there are arguments or stress? That is a good question.

Pregnancy is a time of change for a woman. Physical changes make a woman wonder if her body will ever return to normal again. Sexual changes vary from no interest, to a heightened sexual desire. Emotional changes consist of adapting to surprise swings of mood, including unexpected joy or pain.

Relationships to our own parents alter during pregnancy. Our relationships with friends change, too, because they may have interests other than babies. Later, you may want the baby but dislike the pregnancy, wishing it were over. Your body image may be damaged as you look at nonpregnant women. A near-to-term mother is susceptible to insults and bothered by those endless comments of "Are you still pregnant?" and "Not delivered yet?" Irritable and tired, you wonder if the time will ever end.

Now, you recall, the baby is experiencing your upheaval! The burning question is: Do I have to change how I react to situations in my life? Dr. Lewis Mehl,[28] a speaker at the 1985 Second Pre- and Perinatal Psychology Conference in San Diego, reminded us, "A baby needs to experience the parents' wide range of feelings. This assists in the baby's neurological development."

Each of us handles a wide range of feelings and different levels of stress. I believe an expectant parent will be wise to seek additional help to handle various needs that arise. Make a commitment to yourself to recognize when you are feeling stressed. Discuss with your doctor your need to know that you can call his office and have your call returned if you are overly worried.

Individualized bonding is illustrated by a mother who talked to her baby frequently throughout the pregnancy. This mother made special arrangements with her unborn baby. She would tell the baby, "Look, I have a real tough day ahead of me at this conference. Please have a peaceful day. No kicking and thrashing and tearing around in there!" On return to her office, when all is settled, and all her upheavals are over, her baby takes off and is incredibly active, while she thanks her baby for the cooperation. Some businesswomen take their portable tape players to work so they can play peaceful music. "It's World War III on my desk today," they tell their babies. "So pay no attention to my stress and my activity up here. I'm going to play some peaceful music for you, so have a nice morning." Then they proceed with their responsibilities.

When I carried my first child, I chose to keep on working at my high-pressure job on the night shift in an intensive care unit. To compound my situation, my father died during the first month of my pregnancy. My mother died one week before I gave birth. During my pregnancy, a staff member on our unit committed suicide. All members of the intensive care staff had to come in for group therapy. Those of us on the night shift had to report at 2:00 p.m. This is like asking people who work on the day shift to get out of bed at 2:00 a.m. When I demonstrated some resistance to this, the psychologist leading the group suggested I did not want my baby. I cried for three days in frustration and anger! It cannot surprise you, with the knowledge that chemical imprints can occur, that my daughter has an easy-to-push stress-level button. It is easy for her to create a storm in a teacup, to worry, to become apprehensive, to become tense and bothered.

When you are feeling stressed, keep talking to your baby and keep sharing your life. Take a relaxing walk or read a soothing story. Choose to write in your diary and allow yourself to let the stress go. Some mothers like to color or paint. You may prefer a body massage or to call a friend. Networking and discussing your concerns are always important. Play soothing music or take a nap. If you have patches of apprehension, remember that other pregnant mothers often feel exactly the same way.

Do not let your baby's awareness become a restriction to living. The strains of everyday living cannot be avoided. Simply be aware of the impact of your words and emotional reactions. I know of a number of arguments which are stopped with the phrase, "Not in front of the b-a-b-y!" This is nothing more than using your baby, whether born or unborn, as a shield. If you are aware of how your behavior impacts others, including baby, there will be no special problem created by your pregnancy. Life with your baby will be natural. If an argument develops, try not to fall into enormous guilt feelings about damaging the child's psyche.

Sharing your whole life is a very important step. In the end, pre-birth bonding is more than a method of getting through the nine-month pregnancy. It is the beginning of a way of life and a way of relating to your child. Your baby is ready, willing, and able to receive love from the earliest moment. The giving of love in a real way is established from the outset. Such a life pattern can be transformational for both the baby and you.

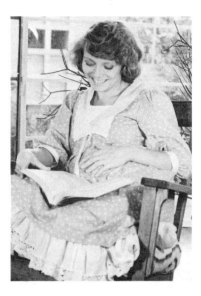

Read to
Your Baby

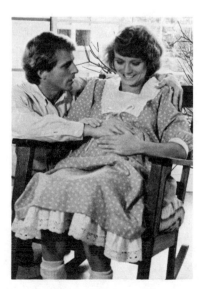

Communicate
with Your Baby

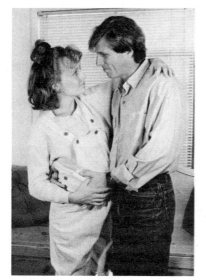

Dance with
Your Baby

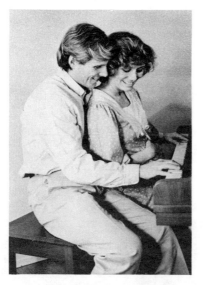

Play Music
for Your Baby

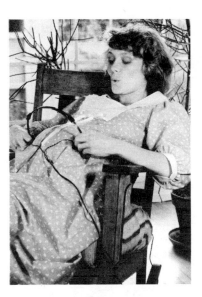

Sing to
Your Baby

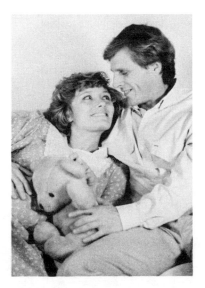

Share Your
Whole Life

6

Visualization

It is one thing to discuss setting aside a time each day to spend with the unborn baby, to relax and to communicate. It is quite another thing to do it. "How do I do that?" you might ask. Communication is the beginning of the relationship. After that first look, or touch, or feeling of acquaintance, you begin to communicate your feelings to the other person. You dream, you daydream, you visualize, and then you take action.

Pre-birth bonding is about more than communication. It is about demonstrating your love, in every practical and conceivable way. This process is a simple reflection of life itself. For what is life, if not a simple demonstration of how you feel, what you think, and what you believe?

The action phase (steps six through ten) comes after the communication phase (steps one through five). After resting, enjoying the baby, making contact, beginning conversation, and learning to share your whole life, you move into the next steps:

6. Visualize

7. Educate Yourself

8. Prepare for the Birth

9. Put Your Plan into Action

10. Experience the Birth

Once you have successully bonded with your baby, you logically decide how you want your life to be with that new family member. This includes how you wish the experience of birth to be.

The sixth step in pre-birth bonding is VISUALIZE. You will use mental picturing techniques to outline what your experiences, including birth, will be with your child.

The following is a transcript of one of my relaxation classes for expectant parents. It is important to be comfortable. I suggest playing peaceful background music while you record the following transcript:

> Make yourself comfortable. You may lie on your side, or lie on your back. With your eyes closed now, breathe out a big sigh, almost breathing right through the middle of your body and out the ends of your feet. Allow yourself to feel really relaxed with your eyes closed and feeling heavy. Notice that you are going along with the rhythm of your own breathing. As you become relaxed, allow your arms to feel heavy, and your legs to feel heavy. Let the tension of the day fall off your body as easily as if you were dropping clothes off a coat hanger onto the floor. Let the tension of the day drop right from your body.
>
> In your mind's eye, allow yourself to recall a beautiful place you have been. This may be on a beach, by the water, in the mountains, by a lake,

or in a garden. When you arrive in this place, notice your beautiful surroundings exactly the way you want them to be. Allow yourself to be totally relaxed at this time. Mothers, rest your hand on your tummy, taking time just to be with your baby. Fathers, rest your hand on the mother's tummy also. Allow yourself to relax. Take time to be with the three of you.

There is nothing special to do, no one to please. You are wonderful beings, taking time out to be with your family. Now, in your mind's eye, put a window on the tummy. Look in and see your beautiful baby. See your baby floating in an amniotic sea. Visualize your baby's soft, downy hair, long eyelashes and fingernails. Notice the occasional smile or hiccup. Observe your baby safe in his world, protected, nurtured, and dependent on you.

Acknowledge yourself for the love, care, and nurturing that brought you to this time. Feel your baby turning, kicking, pulling away, and being still to your touch. Take time to feel and touch your baby each day, time that the baby knows is for a love touch. See your baby exploring his world by touching the cord, the walls of the uterus, and his own limbs.

Understand your baby is exercising his muscles and developing beautifully in readiness for birth. Wonder at what your baby can hear: the internal sounds of your bladder and bowels, the comforting regular sound of your heartbeat, and your blood surging in your blood vessels. Your baby also hears blood returning through the umbilical cord to the placenta. Realize that your baby is learning to breathe and is setting his life rhythms to the beat of these motherly sounds.

Your baby always hears the mother's voice,

responds to the father's voice, and, later, responds to outside sounds.

Stop and pause and remember, "Where have I been? What has my baby been hearing?" Sort out your thoughts about that and send thoughts to your baby. Be open to receive thoughts from the baby. Observe your feelings about the day and share your truth with the baby about those feelings.

Notice that your baby swallows, sucks his thumb, responds to strong lights, and opens and closes his eyes at various times. Your baby is receiving chemical inputs from your various daily activities. If it is appropriate, share mental messages with your baby.

In your mind's eye, see your partner, your doctor, or midwife. Visualize the delivery area when it is known to you. See the nurses, the anesthesiologist, the pediatrician, all of whom you may not know. See your immediate family and friends. This is your network of support that you are creating for your pregnancy, labor, and afterward. Draw white lines connecting these people. These are lines of communication. Know you will open these lines of communication to bring in the information you need to have a good experience, the best possible birthing experience for the three of you. Share your day's activities with your baby as you go about your life. Let your baby know who you are and what you are thinking about this special gift, your baby, whom you nurture and cherish right now in your womb.

As you choose to bring this time with the baby to a close, remember to close the window on your tummy and to bring yourself and the baby back into present time. As you come back into present time, wriggle your toes, stretch, and yawn. Only when you feel comfortable, begin to open your eyes.

This is a guided visualization. It allows you a frame of mind where communication with your baby becomes comfortable, easy, and natural. Visualization is a life-long process. In some quarters it is highly controversial; in others, it is considered the only step necessary to achieve success, happiness, wealth, and joy in every area of your life. It is not unique to pre-birth bonding. It opens up other avenues of communication as well— communication with yourself and your partner. Imagine how life would be if you let your partner know, as I am suggesting you let the baby know: where you are going, what you are doing, why you are doing it, what you are feeling, why you are feeling it, and who you are.

Only by letting others know who we are, can we ever really be ourselves.

Visualization is a strong mental tool. It creates the space or the frame of mind to handle today as well as tomorrow. It can be used to choose how you want things to be. In pre-birth bonding, you use it in a highly focused way to achieve specific results in your life. At this time you are concerned mainly with your baby's birth and the period immediately after. In this step you visualize all the details of the remainder of the preg-nancy: the birth itself, the post-partum, the details of your baby's surroundings, bonding in the delivery room, nursing and feeding, and the early growth period. Let us continue with another visualization transcript used for further relaxation and the birth of the baby.

Again, you are breathing in and out easily, going along with the rhythm of your own breath-ing, choosing again to be in a beautiful place and relaxed. Again, in your mind's eye, picture the three of you and see your relationship to your doctor and how you will work together through the rest of your pregnancy and into labor and delivery. Take some time to do this now, running through the scenario in your mind from today, continuing through your pregnancy into labor, delivery, and afterward. While you listen to the music, visualize the relationship, rest comfortably, and feel relaxed.

I want both the mother and father to tense up your right arms. In your mind's eye, this tense arm represents a contraction. Allow the contraction to be really firm and strong. While you are experiencing the contraction, continue to breathe the same amount of breath easily, and relax the rest of your body around each contraction. Now relax your right arm, experience it as being warm, heavy, and relaxed.

Now tense up your left arm. Again, experience another contraction while you continue to breathe easily, and relax the rest of your body around each contraction. Now relax your left arm. Now tense your right arm and your left leg. This represents two areas of tension, which is quite common at the end of the first stage of labor when the cervix is almost fully dilated. While you are experiencing two areas of tension, continue to breathe easily, be relaxed around the contraction and the tension. Now relax your arm and leg. This gives you the knowledge that you can be relaxed throughout the contractions of your labor.

Notice that when you are relaxed your eyes are heavy, your nostrils are relaxed, your jaw is heavy, and your lips separated as you breathe easily. Your shoulders are heavy and relaxed. Your tummy is bulging and relaxed. Your buttocks are heavy and relaxed. Your legs are so heavy you can barely move them. This deep relaxation can be used between labor contractions to assist you to regain your energies for the next contraction. You may wish to sleep between contractions in labor, as sleeping for a few minutes will seem like a whole night.

In your mind's eye, picture yourself coming into labor. Notice the teamwork involved with your baby, for it is your baby who puts the hormone out that commences labor. So talk to your baby if you go past your due date. Often a baby will respond when the options are explained clearly. When way overdue, some couples have described the joys and beauty of the outside world to their baby. One couple described butterflies and the softness of kittens to encourage the curiosity of their baby to be born. Conversely, you may want to communicate about not coming into a premature labor, explaining to your baby the reasons and benefits of staying in your womb until he is better able to handle breathing in the outside world. Your communication can be clear and precise as though you were talking to another adult. So picture your labor commencing in your mind's eye. Familiarize yourself with the contractions and how they work. Visualize the contractions massaging and stimulating your baby in readiness for the outside world. Imagine your contractions gently opening the cervix, or entrance to the womb; your baby's head pushing up against the cervix, assisting the cervix to open to its maximum stretch. Know that you will adopt positions that will assist you in labor and will support your comfort.

Trust your knowledge of your body to help you adapt to this new experience. You can go into the pain that results from the cervix stretching, knowing that you have the capacity to handle it. Visualize your cervix stretching to the width of the palm of your hand. Continue to see yourselves working peacefully together in preparation for the birth itself.

Once your cervix is fully opened, you can push the baby down and into the birth canal. See your baby molding his head to adapt to the passage. Suggest to your baby that you can work together easily during the birth. Observe your baby coming to the outlet, the vulva, which is a second doorway through which your baby has to be born. Visualize the muscles of your pelvic floor relaxing, stretching, and making way for your baby's molded head. Visualize the top of your baby's head appearing between the vulva and see this outlet gradually stretch as your baby eases through this outlet. Visualize yourself adapting to positions and changes that would support you most for the birth. Imagine the baby being lifted onto your tummy, hear his first cry, and watch your baby opening his eyes. Feel the weight and warmth of your baby resting on your tummy as you reach down to welcome, hold, and caress. Visualize all details of the birth that are important to you. Experience in your mind's eye the incredible joy of giving birth. Think for a few moments about your new family. Think about coming home, starting a life with a new person that you can now see, hold, touch, and enjoy. Continue to picture these things while being very relaxed, and while breathing easily in your own rhythm.

With your thoughts about how you would like the birth to be, breathe out with a big sigh, and gradually allow yourself to come back into this time and space. Always remember to bring your baby with you. Again, wiggle your toes, stretch and yawn, and only when you want to, open your eyes.

There are many books on visualization. It is an astoundingly simple subject. There is nothing really to do, except to use your mind, your imagination, and the picture window of your brain. No one way is better than another. All that is necessary is that you are clear on what you want. This may be difficult in some areas of your life, such as finding the perfect partner or the perfect life's work. You already know what you want with regard to the birth of your baby: an entrance into this world free of complications, a birth that makes your baby feel welcome into this life, and a birth that is comfortable and without unnecessary strain, effort, struggle, or pain.

How does visualization work? This explanation you must take on faith alone, because there seems to be no way to prove it except through results. If you doubt yourself going into the process, then it is not going to work for you. Faith is the key in the visualization process. The only way we know to verify the effectiveness of visualization, other than through individual results, is to talk to people, or read the accounts of people who have used the process to great benefit.

Visualization is one of the simplest, yet most profound, of all the steps. It involves no one but yourself. It can be done at any place, at any time. Often visualization is done before sleeping or just after awakening, when your mind is not cluttered. You can visualize as you go about your daily tasks. In your mind, run through the entire pregnancy. Be deliberate in placing these pictures in your mind exactly the way you want them to be. Add words to the pictures, creating positive statements—called affirmations—which are very powerful.

Visualize at least once a day. Do not worry about unwanted thoughts, such as, "What if there is a problem?" Discard the thought as soon as you have it. I suggest your visualization time be approximately fifteen minutes. Music can help you immensely, relaxing your mind and making it receptive.

Get comfortable in a room or place you find particularly inviting. Relax at the beginning. Keep breathing; it will help you relax. In your mind, begin as if you are watching a movie. Run through the pictures from beginning to end. Start wherever you wish, at the moment you are in now, and right on through the pregnancy. Start at the moment birthing begins, or start at whatever the beginning is for you, and then run your pictures through to the end. Watch these pictures even as you create them. Once you have created the perfect script, or the perfect prayer, run it over and over again each time you visualize. When you have concluded, bring yourself back into the present. Do not do this by simply opening your eyes, but visualize the room you are in and then see yourself in the present moment. Then, when you are ready, open your eyes.

Breathe deeply and notice how relaxed you feel. Visualizing is always relaxing, fulfilling, comforting, and wonderful.

Some time ago I discovered the fascinating story of anthropologist Robbie E. Davis-Floyd, who chose to use visualizations during her pregnancy. Dr. Davis-Floyd has researched, for the last decade, pregnancy and childbirth in the United States. In her dissertation, "Birth as an American Rite of Passage,"[29] she recalls her own experience:

Shortly before I became pregnant with my second child, I read that pregnancy was an ideal time for psychotherapy. With the help of a good therapist, a pregnant woman could accomplish in several months what would usually take several years. Apparently, this is possible because so many things are in flux during a woman's pregnancy. Not only her body, but also her emotions, her lifestyle, and her relationships with herself and her mate and the rest of the world. So, I was determined to take the opportunity offered by my second pregnancy to explore as much of myself as possible.

Visualization seemed a particularly intriguing technique, especially since my first experience with childbirth, a cesarean section, had called into question my whole relationship with my body. It had made me see how disconnected I was. Visualization offered a way for me to pursue that reintegration of body and mind, which I could see was absolutely necessary to birth vaginally this time.

To begin with, I wanted to resolve some fears I had about whether the cesarean scars on my stomach and uterus were strong enough to support the labor and birth of what I felt sure would be a big baby. (I was right, he weighed ten pounds at birth.)

I also wanted to know why my cervix had never dilated past four centimeters after twenty-seven hours of labor and if it could and would dilate this time around. I chose to use my first visualization experience to seek answers to these questions. I was most fortunate to have as my guide Susan McKay, a psychologist, International Childbirth Education Association consultant, and author of *The Assertive Approach to Childbirth*.[30] We were co-participants in a workshop on visualization given by Gayle Peterson and Lewis Mehl.

Susan began by helping me achieve a high degree of relaxation through feeling each part of my body. Then, at her suggestion, I visualized my consciousness as a cell in my bloodstream going down through my body until I came to my cesarean scars. As I gazed at them from the inside, I had the impression of enormous railroad tracks across my skin, which were tremendously strong and durable. I understood that they would hold, no matter how big the baby, and I felt newly confident and reassured. Susan took me deeper, down through my uterus until I gazed at my cervix. I was amazed to see how red, thick, and strong it was. Clearly a most powerful muscle.

Susan suggested that I ask its purpose. I did and received an immediate sense that it was there to hold in and to protect. When I asked why it had never dilated fully during my first labor, I was swept by feelings of tremendous confusion. How could it be expected to hold in and protect one moment and to let go the next?

On the heels of that realization came a strong feeling that more time for the labor plus some mind-body integration could have overcome the confusion. My cervix would have dilated, but something else had stopped it.

Susan took me a little deeper into the altered state, and all of a sudden I was flooded by waves of pain and fear brought about by sharp, long suppressed memories of bright lights, harsh voices, and many hands sticking up inside my cervix and causing me great pain for during that first labor, I was checked for dilation almost every half an hour by various hospital personnel.

As I wept with that newly remembered anguish, I understood that my cervix had remained closed in protective response to my body's overall sense of invasion and danger during labor. This visualization was a very moving experience for both Susan and me.

It was enlightening because it helped me to understand the strength of the subconscious connection between the mind and the body. Having discovered what a potentially powerful and rewarding tool visualization was, I realized that it might offer a way for me to solve the mystery of the nausea that had plagued both my mother and me during each pregnancy. A nausea so severe, that we threw up literally everything we ate. This had caused my mother to miscarry three babies, a fate which I managed to avoid by taking the controversial drug, Bendectin. The drug stopped the nausea completely as long as I took it regularly. I did not like using the Bendectin, but I did not want to throw up twelve or thirteen times a day.

For my second pregnancy, I found a therapist in my home town who was experienced in the use of visualization. After trying several unsuccessful techniques involving my family history, she hit upon the simpler idea of having me ask my stomach, during a visualization, why it continually threw up. My stomach then helped me clearly to understand that it was only following orders and that I ought to ask my brain.

I could not seem to get in touch with my brain, so my therapist had me visualize it as a computer screen. I sat at the keyboard and punched in my question. "What is the source of this nausea?" On the screen appeared the response that the nausea came from an ancient program which originally had to do with the survival of a certain group of people and which had been passed to me and to my mother and me genetically through a great-grandmother.

I thought, "Well great, I'll just cancel the program." But when I typed in a command to cancel, the screen just flashed on and off. I could not get the command to enter. I started to slump in my chair with exhaustion from the tremendous mental effort, but the therapist said, "Hey, this is not supposed to be a battle. Try a gentler approach." So I cancelled the command, the screen stopped flashing, and I typed in: "Why does the Bendectin work?" My brain responded: "It short-circuits the program." I then typed in a new command to substitute vitamin B-6 for Bendectin. (Vitamin B-6 is one of the components of Bendectin and is considered safe for use in pregnancy.) This command was accepted. That night, I went off the Bendectin again (after many unsuccessful prior attempts), but kept taking B-6. I felt slightly nauseated the next day but did not throw up.

By the following day, I had no more nausea at all. I thought that the whole thing was very strange, but what did I care, it had worked. Each time I did a visualization, the process for entering the altered state was slightly different, varying especially with the individual styles of the people guiding me.

The therapist who guided me through most of my visualizations would begin by having me sit in a big, cushy, reclining armchair. I would close my eyes, and she would ask that I relax into the chair, feeling how its soft cushiness supported the weight of my body, my head, my arms, my back, my legs, and feet. She would suggest that I sense each of these, allowing the chair to support that part of me, trusting that I was safe. Then she would have me imagine a golden ball of light hovering right over the top of my head, beautiful and shining. As she spoke, I could see the ball of light begin to melt like warm golden honey, flowing warm and slow down my face, my forehead, my eyelids, my nose, my mouth and chin, my neck, my breasts, etc., until, little by little, I experienced every part of me as glowing with warm, golden light and, thus, was able to come to a strong sense of the unity and totality of my body.

At that point, she would begin the specific suggestion for whatever sort of visualization we had agreed to do that day, and I usually found it easy to take my consciousness down inside my body in such a relaxed state. Sometimes, I would tense up, thinking I wouldn't be able to do it. But my therapist always gave me permission not to try too hard, to "just begin to imagine, without really trying, but just to begin to allow myself to imagine . . ."

My next visualization was truly beautiful. I saw the baby inside my uterus, sleeping peacefully with its head resting on the placenta as if it were a pillow. I began by visualizing myself as a tiny, little person standing on my own face. Then walking into my nose and heading down toward my stomach. The therapist had me visualize a window in my uterus, through which I could see the baby. Finally, I was able to step through the window and onto the baby's foot. I walked along his leg, past his genitals. I could see clearly that he was a boy. When I got to his chest, I could see his face and his closed eyes.

I called to him and he cocked one sleeping eye. I asked, feeling a little silly, if he would help me give birth to him vaginally. I received the very clear response that he was not disposed to worry about what might, or might not, happen in three months. His reality was totally in the here and now; the here and now was very beautiful and peaceful, and I should just relax! He went back to sleep and I took my departure, feeling duly chastened, but tremendously pleased and reassured.

I felt ready to tackle the memory of my cesarean birth experience. I wanted to heal and clear that experience so that I would not subconsciously try to repeat, as people often do, when they have not worked something through. (See *Birthing Normally*.[31]) For me, the most painful part of the cesarean had been not being allowed to watch my daughter's birth.

After twenty-seven hours of total involvement with my body, I had been horrified to lose not only physical, but also visual, contact with my body. There had been no way for me to participate in her birth as a person, and in my own birth as a mother. I had begged the doctor to let me watch. His refusal left me feeling weak, irrelevant, and helpless, feelings which stayed with me and kept surfacing in various ways.

In my healing visualization, I rewrote all these messages. As the green curtain descended, separating me from my lower body, I began to talk to the doctor. This time I gathered all my personal power and used it to convince the doctor to overcome his medical school training and move the green curtain, allowing my face to be inside the sterile field, wearing a mask like everyone else in the room.

Holding my husband's hand, I watched my daughter's birth with fascination, at least as much of it as I could see over the huge mound of my stomach. I hadn't even realized that my belly would block part of the view until I was actually visualizing it! I saw the doctor lift the baby out, all covered with vernix and blood. He handed her straight to me and I held her, just as I had wanted to, and was absolutely overjoyed.

It's amazing, but the memory of that visualization is just as real to me as the memory of the actual operation. I feel that I lived both, and I feel healed of the grief that I lived with for so long. It seems, after all, that we can rewrite the past. This possibility could prove especially valuable in healing grief from the death of someone you love and were not able to say goodbye to, or perhaps the grief of a terrible mistake you made and feel you will never be able to correct.

The last visualization I did during pregnancy was right around my due date. We had moved from Chattanooga, Tennessee to Austin, Texas. I didn't know any therapists in Austin, so I asked a friend, Rima Star, author of *The Healing Power of Birth*,[32] who is experienced in rebirthing to serve as my guide.

For the last few weeks, the baby had been posterior, that is, with the back of his head toward my back, instead of toward my front. I knew that he would have to turn soon if he was going to, and I wanted to encourage his turning because the posterior position often makes for a more difficult labor. As soon as I felt I had contact with the baby, I received a clear sense of distress involving the umbilical cord.

I got worried because I couldn't seem to visualize him clearly enough to find out what the problem was. I felt stuck, but Rima encouraged me to breathe more deeply and smoothly, using the kind of breathing that is done in rebirthing.

After several minutes of breathing, I could see the baby clearly. It was as if my consciousness was in the womb with him, and I saw that his head was deeply engaged in my pelvis. The cord went from the placenta across the back of his neck and over his left shoulder down to his navel. He was afraid that if he turned anterior, the cord would cut across his throat and choke him, since he could no longer slip it over his head.

We stayed with this sense of fear for awhile, until Rima had the idea that he could take hold of the cord and just slip it down off his left shoulder after he turned. I made this suggestion to him, and received an immediate sense of acceptance and relief. Soon after that he did turn, and was born one week later, tightly holding the cord with both hands, just below his left shoulder.

As I stated at the beginning of this, psychotherapeutic techniques can be particularly rewarding during pregnancy, because this is always a time of psychological upheaval. As the body changes, so must old habits and thought patterns change to include new life.

The experience of growing a baby inside, as well as mothering a newborn, puts women in much closer touch with their own childhood experiences, allowing old, deeply buried thoughts and emotions to surface. Hopes, aspirations, and fears from the past and for the future merge at the surface of daily consciousness, as time contracts in the physical experience of pregnancy, and past, present, and future together are carried in the mother's womb.

I knew about these things when I began my second pregnancy. I knew I had tremendous amounts of fear and grief, and many years of mental alienation from my body, that needed to be healed and released from their lodging places. So I consciously chose to make the best possible use of the opportunities offered by the...pregnancy.

It is my hope that this story of my experiences with visualization may inspire others to incorporate this rewarding technique into their own quests for self-discovery and personal growth.

Dr. Davis-Floyd's personal experience provides a wonderful example of how visualization supports birth in very positive ways. You may wish to visualize with a psychologist or a person experienced in visualization techniques, to support you through uncomfortable memories.

There is no value in beating yourself up over what you experience. It is all right, for instance, to experience morning sickness as your body adapts to the pregnancy. Think about how your body is changing. Look inward for things to do to support the changes. Your mind will lead the way.

Often, your mind communicates unconscious thoughts or ideas to you through dreams. Dreams were uncharted territory for me until I attended Dr. Patricia Maybruck's presentation on dreams at the 1987 International Childbirth Education Association (ICEA) conference. Through subsequent correspondence with Dr. Maybruck and by reading her doctoral dissertation, "An Exploratory Study of Pregnant Women's Dreams,"[33] I became interested in ways dreams could help in prebirth bonding.

I suggested in a discussion with my colleagues, "Pregnant women, pay attention to your dreams." Pat Granados, a childbirth educator, who was pregnant with her sixth child, shared with me her story about her dreams. She had a recurring dream about waking up in a pool of blood with her baby delivered. She followed up by having a sonogram which showed that the placenta (her afterbirth) was in the normal position, on the upper section of her uterus. Her dream occurred early in the pregnancy and was repeated exactly the same way. Pat began taking time to be with her baby, talking and visualizing what was going on in her uterus.

It seemed clear to Pat that her baby was going to be born early, so she kept telling her baby, "You must wait until the thirty-sixth week" (when her baby would be more likely to handle breathing in the outside world). She spent considerable time talking to her baby about developing perfectly and she visualized a normal birth.

Pat came into labor on the thirty-sixth week by trickling a pool of blood. Her dream was accurate. Her placenta had separated on one edge, and she was bleeding internally. There was some consideration about doing a cesarean section. However, in a very short space of time, she delivered a normal, healthy baby girl, whose breathing was perfect, and who had no need to go into intensive care. A month or so after her delivery, I saw Pat and she said to me, "You saved my baby's life." I said, "No, you paid attention to the dream!"

Sheila Kitzinger, anthropologist, and in my opinion, probably the greatest writer and contributor to childbirth today, wrote about dreams in *Your Baby, Your Way*:[34] "Sometimes, tracking dreams down and recollecting them can help to pinpoint anxiety, which has been unacknowledged. It is often useful to do this so that something can be done to defuse the anxiety."

You may want to jot down any pregnancy dreams you feel throw some light on your hopes and fears, and on things that are important to you about the birth and the baby.

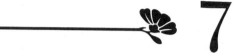

Education

With each step in pre-birth bonding you move closer to the perfect birth and the perfect life for you and your child. This process sets up things the way you want them to be.

Step seven in pre-birth bonding is EDUCATE YOURSELF. Of course, the whole bonding process is one of education, but in this step you focus on the specific results you want to achieve. You have learned to visualize and now you want to become specific about what pictures you place on the screen of your mind. You may not know at this stage exactly what you want with regard to the birth of your child. Education will assist you in finding out.

All steps in pre-birth bonding take time and commitment. So, I urge you to set aside a specific amount of time each day for self-education. It might be the last thirty minutes to an hour before going to sleep. It might be a fifteen minute period in the middle of your day. It might be the time between the onset of early morning activity and the noon rush.

Pick the perfect time and stick to it. Do not waiver and do not renege on your commitment. Use this time everyday to educate yourself. The length of time you spend is not nearly as important as spending this time daily. Ten to fifteen minutes every day can add up to a lot of education in a month.

The purpose of this step is to focus on the whole wonderful experience of childbirth and see, really, what it is all about, and what it can mean for you. Educating yourself can be valuable even for those who have had several children and think they have seen it all. There are alternatives arising every day.

Education begins by your decision to learn, or to learn anew, all you possibly can about bonding, birthing, and parenting. This means researching and reading about life and birth. It means listening. A basic reading program is essential. This is where the fifteen to twenty minutes each day come in. Put together a reading list of magazines and books. Commit yourself to reading this material a little each day over the entire term of your pregnancy. (See the Suggested Reading in the Appendix.)

Learn how to pick the perfect doctor for you. Learn about alternative birthing centers. Learn about L.D.R.'s (labor, delivery, and recovery rooms), which are sometimes called family birth units. Learn of new techniques in childbirth. As you study these things, you can draw a clearer picture of how you want the birth of your child to proceed, exactly what you want to happen and how you want it to happen. Then you create your visualization from a firm base. You will know the mental pictures you want to create.

After setting up your reading program, begin to scan the television program listings to see what television has to offer. You will be surprised at the number of telecasts—especially on public television—that deal with childbirth issues. Video rentals are another source of childbirth preparation movies. Scan your local newspaper for lectures in your area. Often lectures are offered for a nominal fee by doctors, nurses, midwives, and others who sincerely want to inform the public about childbirth and childbirth alternatives. Take your partner and go to the lectures. Listen carefully and ask questions. As you collect information that will enable you to choose a doctor, a hospital, a general practitioner, or a midwife, remember that there is no such thing as a question you cannot ask. When it comes to the birth of your child, there needs to be no question unanswered, no concern unaddressed, no fear unresolved, no personal desire unfulfilled. It is amazing, but true, that many people pay more attention, ask more questions, get more answers, and look more closely at every aspect of buying a car or leasing an apartment than they do having a child. This is the most important single event in the life of your child. Yet, some people plan more for their child's first birthday or for the baby's first Christmas than they do for the baby's birth.

One good source of information about birth is new mothers. Go to a park, admire a newborn, and then say, "Do you have a few minutes to tell me about your delivery? What was it really like? Would you have done anything differently?" These mothers are an immediate source of information about how deliveries are being handled in your community. Some new mothers will tell you about their relaxed obstetrician who gave them space to experience birth in their own manner. Others will tell you about doctors who had to control every step of the process.

Recently a newly pregnant mother called me to say she had received information on nutrition from her doctor. However, included in the packet were several pages of disclaimers. These forms, that the mother was requested to sign, relieved the doctor of any responsibility regarding the birth. The mother did not feel comfortable with the lengthy disclaimer which was mailed in such an impersonal manner and not discussed with her, so she switched to another obstetrician.

Becoming acquainted with birth is, like bonding,

done step by step. In the rigorously clinical, medicated deliveries done in modern hospitals, it is increasingly rare to have a natural delivery. You might look at the issue of safe birthing in different settings: in hospitals with a physician attending, at home with a physician, or at home with a lay-midwife attending.

Another good subject to learn about is labor and delivery positions. Janet Isaacs Ashford, who produced a quarterly magazine, *Childbirth Alternatives*, has collected 500 pictures of women, in every culture and age in the history of humankind, giving birth in an *upright* position. It is not common knowledge that women naturally gave birth in this manner.

The first time I became aware of the history of birthing was in the early 1980s when Dr. Michel Odent gave a talk at a conference in San Francisco. Dr. Odent said that women now lie down on their backs, with their feet stuck up in the air, to give birth, all because of the French King Louis XIV, who wanted to watch his mistress deliver. The King's doctor obliged him by putting the woman on her back and cutting a hole in the delivery room wall so the King could observe.

This does not mean a delivery in an upright position is preferred. You may choose to be upright during the second stage of labor in order to bring the baby's head down onto the muscles of your pelvic floor. You may, in fact, choose numerous positions: to stay upright, to lie on your side, or to use one of the new birthing beds which supports a squatting position and provides a bar to hold onto. Alternatively, you could be on your hands and knees, or deliver in water. (But, when the time comes to deliver, you may not feel that any particular position is of importance.)

An upright position will hasten the labor because of the pressure against the cervix. This may become uncomfortable and so you may choose, in early labor, to lie down for fifteen minutes every hour, or to sit. Also in early labor, you can walk, take showers, rest, and sit on the toilet facing the back, resting your head on a pillow on the tank. You may find that laboring is more comfortable on your hands and knees. Lean on walls, the backs of chairs, against your partner, or other support persons. Surround yourself with only loving supportive people. Do everything possible to avoid going to bed and making labor an illness. Do not feel it is necessary to be in bed. Sometimes lying on your side may give you needed time to rest, and frequently it is the best position for blood flow to the baby. Before insisting on any position, check with the person monitoring the birth to be certain the position is safe for you and your baby.

As labor proceeds, time your contractions and keep in touch with your obstetrician. Ask ahead of time when to call her and when to go to the hospital. This is extremely important because, first, she knows your obstetric history and, second, she knows the distance you must travel to the delivery facility. Never drive your vehicle while you are in labor! Contractions may cause you to floorboard the accelerator. Devise another plan to reach the birth facility if your partner is not around.

When the labor becomes intense, sitting in warm water is an excellent place to be. When you lie down on the bed, turn on your side as much as possible to take weight off the large blood vessels in your pelvis, so that oxygen to your baby is not reduced.

If it is necessary for your delivery to use a modern medical facility with wires, an intravenous, electronic monitors, blood pressure cuffs, etc., you will need to call the nurse so you can move around. I strongly urge you to keep doing just that, for that is what the staff is for.

Read books on childbirth preparation. Take the classes, see the movies, and make your plans for positions to use in labor. Practice, practice, and practice in all the positions so labor becomes second nature to you when the time comes. Remember, you can always change your mind about anything at any time.

The new birthing beds in modern hospitals are adjustable. Make sure, however, that the nurse taking care of you knows how to maneuver the bed into the various positions you may want.

Recently, when I was demonstrating birthing positions to a class, I explained that women used to lean on tree trunks during the second stage of labor. I developed the giggles. I visualized us transporting trees into the labor and delivery area. The more I thought about it, the more I giggled. Soon, ten couples and I were laughing uproariously. Two thoughts come from this story. First, trees would be delightful in the delivery area. Second, you cannot be tense while you are laughing! So remember to use your sense of humor as a tool during your labor.

Another time, I coached a woman during a lengthy labor which was being filmed. She had chosen to labor naked. About four in the morning, after twelve hours of labor, she leaned against her husband's back in the bed, looked up at the cameraman and between contractions casually said, "Your fly is undone." He replied, "*You* should talk!" We all laughed for a long time after these exchanges.

Laughter can be very healing, because it releases important chemicals into your body. So, put laughter on your list; it will serve you well.

Cesarean section (surgical incision of the walls of the abdomen and uterus to deliver) is another subject to pursue. For example the headline to an article by Dan Sperling in *USA Today*, November 3, 1987, read, "Needless Surgery." On the same day, a headline in the *San Diego Union* read, "C-Sections Unnecessary in Half 1986 Cases, Group Says." The article was written from a report by Ralph Nader. An article in the *Los Angeles Times*, November 19, 1987, called "C-Sections, Are

There Too Many?" cited the Hospital Council of Southern California's expressed concern about consumers misinterpreting raw data in terms of quality care. Hospitals with a high rate of cesarean sections in Southern California are A.M.I. of Tarzana (in Los Angeles), with a 39.1 percent rate; Coastal Community Hospital in Santa Ana, with a 33.9 percent rate; and Scripps Memorial Hospital in La Jolla, with a 37.6 percent rate.

Some hospitals, including large, academically affiliated medical centers that deliver many high-risk babies, have strong cesarean section control programs. The rates for these hospitals are: UCLA Medical Center, with 16.4 percent; Martin Luther King, Jr.-Drew Medical Center, with 13.3 percent; Kaiser Hospital of Anaheim, with 16.8 percent; and the Naval Regional Medical Center in San Diego, with 12.2 percent.

Whatever the form of delivery, your goal is a healthy baby and there are many excellent reasons for a cesarean section. Discuss these with your obstetrician. Do not valiantly put yourself through endless hours of labor if cesarean section is indicated.

I think it is important for you to know that in the United States there is about a 30 percent chance of having a cesarean section birth in the hospital. A study in the *New England Journal of Medicine*,[35] February 12, 1987, revealed sharp differences in cesarean section rates among nineteen industrial countries. In 1981, these differences ranged from a low of fifty per thousand hospital deliveries in Czechoslovakia to a high in the United States of 180 per thousand hospital deliveries. The study also details—from among a wide range of data on obstetric practices—the percentage of mothers who had a vaginal delivery after a previous cesarean (5 percent of the mothers giving birth in the United States, as compared to 43 percent in Norway, where the cesarean section rate was one-half of that in the United States).

Although the American Medical Association reports a cesarean section rate of 33 percent in California, the rate varies from doctor to doctor. Some doctors have a much higher cesarean section rate than others.

I believe monitoring and fear are two of the major contributing factors to prolonged labor, which leads to a high percentage of cesarean sections. The fear which produces adrenaline, and prolongs labor, was studied by Dr. Caldeyro-Barcia[36] of South America. He observed in a herd of animals that when fear was present a laboring mother would continue to have strong contractions which produced no results. As the herd moved and the fear dissipated, the laboring mother would continue in a normal fashion to a productive labor.

In the event you find the dilation of your cervix stuck for several hours at a certain point, for example four centimeters, you may be heading into a prolonged labor. Before accepting Pitocin, a drug to strengthen your contractions, try these suggestions:

- relaxing with music and visualization techniques,

- resting and sleeping,

- showering,

- getting up and walking around,

- leaning on a wall,

- dimming the lights, and

- reducing all stimulation.

Discuss the situation with the baby. And consider the possibility of making love (the prostaglandins present in semen stimulate labor). This practice may be introduced in the modern hospital setting with its private birthing rooms. The shower is often a wonderful place to make love. Ina May Gaskin,[37] an advocate of natural childbirth and head midwife at "The Farm," a childbirth center in Summertown, Tennessee, recommends to couples when in this tense state of no progress, to go into the forest and make love.

Sometimes, despite all your attempts to relax, nothing works. When this happens, modern medicine provides many options. Be prepared to make an adjustment; it will seem like modern technology is taking over. At first all the procedures may make you feel restricted and tied to the bed. You can proceed with the Pitocin, an intravenous drip with a pump attached, an automatic blood pressure cuff (which makes a beep and may tend to scare you until you are used to it), and constant fetal monitoring.

When electronic fetal monitoring came into existence in the 1960s, it was hailed as the biggest safety-increasing factor in childbirth in a century. Though still widely used, its efficacy is now in question. In my opinion, fetal monitoring is useful (it does save babies' lives, but its negative aspects are devastating),[38] however, even with 100 percent fetal monitoring, your baby can still be born "gray," or need rescuing. Therefore, I do not recommend relying completely on this piece of equipment.

One problem with electronic monitoring is the machine itself. The medical personnel in the room tend to ignore the mother and become hooked on the equipment. Another negative aspect with the monitor is the mother's inability to move around easily. When the mother changes position, the nurse may rush to say, "You moved." The mother's adrenaline goes up, and she becomes subservient to the equipment, the nurse, and the thwarted process. The rise of adrenaline, in turn, is a great detriment to labor. Thus, monitoring may prolong labor and lead to a long series of interventions, including drugs to stimulate labor, pain killers, an epidural anesthetic, forceps, or cesarean section.[39]

Health practitioners such as myself like to check to see how your baby is handling labor. So we listen to the baby's heart rate and monitor progress intermittently. Ten to fifteen minutes an hour is a good compromise, with the understanding that you can be monitored more in the event there are changes on the monitoring strip which indicate your baby may not be tolerating labor well.

Studies have shown that monitoring increases cesarean section deliveries, which carry three times the risk of death, presumably because doctors act on misinterpreted data. Monitors can show false signs of fetal distress as often as 77 percent of the time. Abnormal fetal heart rates can disappear when the mother changes position, usually from lying on her back to lying on her side or sitting upright. Other studies have shown that it is best for many women in labor to be walking around freely. An improvement is the microchip monitor, currently in development, which allows the mother to be monitored while she is moving about.

It is commonly thought that labor speeds up when the doctor artificially ruptures the membranes lining the uterus. Although this procedure may speed up labor by twenty minutes, there are serious drawbacks. The water cushion was put there by nature for a good reason, to protect your baby's head.

Dr. Roberto Caldeyro-Barcia,[40] who has researched this procedure, does not feel it is justified. He cites studies which show that the baby's head suffers from the rupturing of the uterine membranes. Without the water, the baby's head receives uneven pressure which affects the alignment of the skull. The longer the water is intact, the better.

Naturally breaking membranes may be the first sign that true labor is imminent. If your "water has broken" and you are at term, that is, ready to deliver, you will come into labor on your own. For those women who do not naturally commence having contractions, the use of nipple stimulation may encourage the onset of contractions. Your health care professional can provide guidelines for using this technique.

Acupressure and acupuncture also can induce contractions. (This is a whole subject of its own, and one which you need to research ahead of time and discuss with your obstetrician.) I recommend using your own judgment, however, and seeking medical intervention only when absolutely necessary.

Talk to your baby. Discussing the situation with the baby has worked wonderfully well for couples I have worked with who have been under pressure to produce contractions and labor. The baby may be able to speed things along. Inducing labor, following ruptured membranes, is not an urgent necessity. You have the right to say "no" to chemical induction. However, infection rates increase dramatically after membranes are ruptured. The risks of nonintervention versus possible infection must be considered by an informed professional.

(When the membranes are ruptured, the mother's temperature is taken frequently to check that no infection is commencing. Vaginal examinations are kept to a minimum. So parents have many choices and much to learn prior to making decisions about how to proceed if this happens.)

Pain is another subject about which there are many aspects and there is much to learn. All of us are sensitive to pain. We experience pain at different levels. Our tolerance to pain is varying and many times we forget that babies feel pain, too.

In November 1987, the *New England Journal of Medicine* published an article[41] on pain in the fetus and newborn by Doctors K.J. Anand and P.R. Hickey, anesthesiologists at Harvard Medical School. They

documented the fact that in utero and thereafter babies
are equipped to experience pain. Babies clearly demonstrate physical and emotional reactions to indicate when
they are having pain. The doctors concluded that
anesthetics ought to be considered for all invasive procedures and that "humane considerations should apply as
forcefully to the care of neonates and young nonverbal
infants as they do to children and adults in similar painful and stressful situations."

The doctors from Harvard have contributed valuable information to all future parents facing decisions
regarding any surgical procedure involving their babies.
They make it easier for expectant parents to look at
birth from the baby's point of view. They cast new light
on the question, "Is birth painful for the baby?" The
epidural anesthetic relieves pain for the mother, but
what about the baby? This question remains open.

The persistence of one mother, Jill Lawson,
prompted the American Academy of Pediatrics to pub-
lish a resolution in September 1987 stating that babies
need to be properly anesthetized when undergoing surgery. An article discussing the issue of operating on
babies without the use of anesthetic appeared in *Insight*
on February 8, 1988.

Aside from surgical procedures now being per-
formed on newborn babies, what about operations per-
formed in utero? (Examples include unblocking a kidney
stone or relieving pressure on the brain.) This surgery is
done with the best of life-saving intentions and is per-
formed with the highest skill available. Scientifically, we
know that in utero a baby responds to its skin surface
being touched at eight weeks into the pregnancy. Via
ultrasound, we see babies pull away from needles
inserted to withdraw samples of the fluid in which the
babies float. Consider the baby and his possible pain
when contemplating surgery, especially in light of the
report from Harvard.

Circumcision pain is another reality for parents to consider. There is no longer medical justification for the procedure. It is inhuman to cut off a piece of very sensitive tissue with no reason, no warning, and no pain relief. If you decide to proceed with circumcision, I suggest that you explain the procedure to your baby. Ask the doctor to use a local anesthetic, and stay with your baby through the surgery. (Dr. David Cheek has found that Jewish men recall circumcision as a "celebration," indicating that emotions play a significant part in the memory of an event.)

Today, epidural anesthetics are frequently used to ease the pain of delivery for mothers. The epidural consists of a small tube inserted into the lower back, outside the sac of spinal fluid. Small doses of numbing medication are given periodically as needed. The tube that is inserted is flexible, and the mother may sit up, or move around the bed during labor. Epidurals have become more refined over the years. Once the mother was numbed from the level of insertion to her toes. Today the affected area may be restricted to the pelvis, so often the mother can still push her baby out.

But there are other drawbacks. With the use of the epidural, approximately 50 percent of babies are unable to rotate themselves and delivery can only be achieved by the use of forceps or by vacuum extractor. Use of forceps requires an episiotomy (a cut made at the time of delivery to enlarge the stretching of the pelvic floor area), which means more pain for the mother and more drugs for the baby. I have a concern for your baby being left to experience birth alone. Cut off from the mother, who is pain-free, providing the epidural works, the baby is left to handle any pain alone.

In February 1988, the International Childbirth Education Association (ICEA) published a critical paper on epidurals.[42] They do not recommend them, yet some of you will deliver in hospitals, where 80 percent of women receive epidurals. You can write for a copy of this evaluation of epidurals.

I question relieving the mother's pain with the epidural and then, with no preparation, suddenly turning it off and allowing her to experience the full thrust of labor. Once the epidural has been turned off, it takes approximately twenty to thirty minutes for pain relief to be re-established. Again, this is another subject that requires discussion with your obstetrician.

In *Birth Reborn*,[43] Michel Odent reports that in France, women who chose to use no medication and were free to follow their own instincts often labored on their hands and knees in early labor, or in warm water, as the labor progressed. Dr. Odent, who has spent over twenty-five years observing birthing mothers, encourages women to give birth in a supported, squatting position.

Giving birth is considered by some to be a sexual event. If you could observe these mothers giving birth, you would hear a loud cry as the baby's head emerges. In this final birthing moment, it is a cry that matches the peak of orgasm.

Keeping your sense of humor intact, consider that we do not need an epidural in order to conceive babies or to enjoy sex! At the moments of orgasm and birth, we are filled with wonderful endorphins. Endorphins are one of many neurohormones, self-made chemicals that are similar to morphine. When you are laboring, your endorphin level rises to combat stress; the same thing happens when you exercise. So we have natural hormones assisting mother and baby in labor. Some mothers appear to be in an altered state in labor—an excellent place for the mother to be. The baby during labor is also producing endorphins. Hence, labor can leave you both feeling exhilarated.

Endorphins decrease when the mother produces adrenaline as a result of fear. The "fight or flight" syndrome may be stimulated by people or events in the laboring area. Inner fears may be stirred up as the labor strengthens. Good support, a quiet atmosphere, and warm showers may assist the mother in returning to a productive labor.

Pushing, or the second stage of labor, is another part of birth that requires good management and discussion with your obstetrician.

When I serve as a labor coach, I like to use the words, "Get behind your baby and gently ease your baby out." I generally whisper these words in the mother's ear. Sheila Kitzinger[44] prefers the use of the word *open* around this stage of labor.

I want to state categorically that you *will* give birth. Birthing is a natural phenomenon. Even if you were paralyzed from the neck down, your baby would still be pushed out by the contracting uterus (unless some physical reason prevents this from occurring). During labor, the muscles of the uterus shorten with each contraction, making the container smaller. In the first stage of labor, the pressure of the contractions cause your baby to be pushed up against the cervix or entrance to the womb. This pressure gradually opens your cervix.

In the second stage of labor, the birthing phase, your baby is pushed down the vagina until the baby's head is pushed up against the pelvic floor. Gradually, this perineal area stretches and the baby's head appears through the vulva. If the perineal stretching occurs very quickly, you will experience a burning sensation. I am adamant that this pushing phase of labor not be turned into a football cheering match, with the birthing staff turning purple and pushing the baby out also. This is totally unnecessary.

When your baby's head crowns, that is, appears through the vulva, it is a wonderful time for you to reach down and touch your baby's head. You may need the permission and assistance of the medical staff to do this, so that they can be prepared to restore the necessary sterile environment for the safety of the baby and yourself.

When you do touch the top of your baby's head, a wonderful smile will cross your face and you will totally relax the pelvic outlet, for when your jaw is relaxed, so is your pelvic floor. This will assist in the birthing of your baby.

To gain that extra centimeter necessary for birthing, you may have to change your position to squatting, being upright, or getting on your hands and knees. Do whatever it takes. The chapter, "Autonomous Birth," in Sheila Kitzinger's *Your Baby, Your Way*,[45] will give you useful information on this subject.

Discuss with your obstetrician the time he will allow from the full dilation of the cervix until birth occurs. For again, this is an area requiring your understanding, your education, and your decision.

Episiotomy is done, on average, 60 to 99 percent of the time in hospital deliveries. One primary reason given for this type of cut is to shorten the second stage, which is the pushing, birthing stage of labor. The other primary reason is to prevent damage to the newborn, and to prevent tearing, especially third degree tears which go into the rectal tissue. Surprisingly, there are few studies in the medical community to justify this routine procedure. One study in 1987, conducted by four doctors in the U.S., found that women who had episiotomies had the *worst* tears. They reevaluated the practice of using them routinely.

The World Health Organization does not recommend routine episiotomies. Doctors Stephen B. Thacker and David H. Banta[46] studied 350 books and articles written from 1860 to 1980 and concluded that arguments for the widespread use of episiotomy do not stand up to scientific scrutiny. In addition, they say that the risks of episiotomy have been largely ignored. Risks are serious tearing, blood loss, pain, infection, and pain when resuming sex.

To reduce the likelihood of episiotomy, Drs. Thacker and Banta suggest perineal massage, warm oil, warm compresses, and a little more time to stretch the perineal floor to allow the baby to birth. If an episiotomy is required, they observe that a midline cut seems to cause less pain in the healing process than a cut to the side. When I talk to women who gave birth before we began using hospitals for birthing, the mothers use the expression, "I ripped and healed." Doctors seem to confirm this healing ability of the body by suggesting that it is more important to bring the *underlying* tissue carefully together than to draw the *surfaces* tightly together. Mother Nature does very good healing work on the human body. Also, local anesthetic given to make the episiotomy less painful is absorbed quickly by the baby. Discuss with your doctor the need for episiotomy.

In choosing a teacher for childbirth preparation in the United States, there are some national organizations which train, teach, and certify their instructors. Such organizations are the American Society of Psychoprophylaxis in Obstetrics (Lamaze), International Childbirth Education Association, and the Childbirth Education Association. These organizations have profound doctrines of childbirth education. Yet, the freedom to teach them is restricted by the specific hospital's policy and the chief obstetrician's personal policy. As you proceed through this learning process, questions to keep in mind are: Is there new information? Has it been researched? Is this hospital policy? Is this the teacher's personal opinion? These same questions apply to practices within the hospital system. Sometimes, hospital staff members will do things for your benefit that may not be the hospital's current policy, because the policy lags behind the latest reading and researching.

Women who choose to be responsible, informed, educated, and to use their own personal power, have great experiences around birth. The birth may not necessarily go the way they planned, but the process is healing for them. The end result is a beautiful, incredible baby who has joined your life.

Education is the vital seventh step in pre-birth bonding. Take advantage of the classes, the lectures, the literature, and the videos and telecasts. Continue to talk to your doctor at length, leaving no stone unturned. With such education, you will use the previous step of visualization more effectively, and you will move to the next step, PREPARE FOR THE BIRTH, more efficiently.

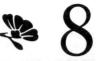

Preparation

PREPARE FOR THE BIRTH is the eighth step in pre-birth bonding. In a sense, the whole process is preparation, and yet, in this step it is meant in a far more specific way. In this step, you will prepare for the birth of your baby right down to the last detail.

During step six, we took a long, measured look at how you wanted the birth to be. We do this step in a quiet, almost meditative state, called visualization. Step seven refined the pictures with education. This gives a clear picture of how you want to give birth and where. In step eight, we prepare to turn your visualizations into reality by making lists, selecting goals, and making decisions. Begin making a list of these goals. Turn your visualizations into reality by writing down how you want it to be.

Birth plans are lists of details that are important to you about birth. Since the beginning of the 1980s, much argument has raged around birth plans. The initial reaction was that birth plans would bother the medical profession. Mothers could not mention such things. The pendulum has swung the other way now, and you will find doctors and obstetric nurses asking for your birth plan to see how they can support you during birth.

Your doctor may be delighted that you want to be informed, happy to discuss her normal routines, and supportive in the outcome of your baby's birth. Your relationship with your birthing support team, including your doctor, is very special and will be developed carefully by you throughout the pregnancy.

In the United States, doctors work under rigorous conditions of frequent lawsuits and horrendous insurance rates. You and I simply would not tolerate these conditions in our job, nor would we wish to continue working under such circumstances. Choose your doctor wisely. Believe that your doctor is doing the very best that he can and would never intentionally harm you. Trust your choice, your intuition, enjoy and make friends with your obstetrician or midwife.

The idea behind birth plans is to have no surprises. During the birth of my first child, I was certainly surprised by having an unfamiliar doctor, a spinal injection, and wrist restraints. The outcome is for you to be informed, to rest assured, knowing that your partner can be present for a cesarean section if he wishes to be, or that you and your partner can accompany your baby to the intensive care nursery if it is necessary for your baby to go there.

Understand that your doctor has a personal life and may not be available when you are ready to give birth, so take time to meet other doctors in the group who may take over for your doctor.

Choose a doctor who will listen to you. I swore after my first delivery, "The next time I deliver, I will choose a doctor who will listen." I did just that. I wanted to use the A.B.C. (Alternative Birthing Center) room. (The A.B.C. room is a room similar to your bedroom at home. It is the hospital's way of giving a more home-like atmosphere for a delivery. Usually the mother does not use an epidural in this room.) I took the obligatory class and forty mothers were in attendance. "Gosh," I thought, "There are not forty days in a month. How will I ever get to use the room?" I started questioning every new mother in the doctor's waiting room. I heard all the reasons under the sun why they were not able to use the A.B.C. room, reasons such as: Someone else was in it. There was not enough staff. It was not clean. It was not ready to use.

I approached the doctor about my thoughts: I could not find anyone who had used the A.B.C. room. I was concerned that I would not get to use it either. My obstetrician heard me. Late in my pregnancy, when my cervix was soft and ready for delivery, my doctor, checking that the room was empty, examined my cervix and ran his finger around the edge, stripping the membrane a little. Sure enough, four hours later I was in labor, in the A.B.C. room. The obstetrician orchestrated a natural delivery. He brought classical music. He directed the photography. He encouraged my husband to take our child's head in his hands once delivered and proceeded with the delivery by lifting Barbara onto my tummy and into my arms. (At this point in delivery, you may reach down and lift your baby onto your tummy yourself.)

My doctor assisted in profound bonding between my husband and baby by touching. All expectant parents could benefit from reading Dr. Ashley Montagu's book, *Touching*,[47] to understand the incredible value and importance of skin-to-skin contact. At delivery you can pull your shirt or gown up over your breasts so that your baby can be placed directly on your skin. Some obstetricians deliberately push your gown up in order to give skin-to-skin contact.

There is nothing preventing the father—provided your baby is in good condition after delivery—from also experiencing skin-to-skin contact with his child. After all, the warm blankets and wrappings provided by hospitals can be put around the parent holding the baby. Skin contact is an event that nurses and hospital staff may support and encourage.

In preparation for developing your birth plan, you may brainstorm what the event of birth means to you and your partner. Birth may mean one or more of the following:

- a physical event

- an emotional event

- a spiritual event

- a healing event

- a legal event

- a birthday

- an event of joy and celebration

- a transitional event

- a sexual event

- a romantic, poetic event

- a family event

Having brainstormed a list of this kind with groups of couples, I have asked, "Well, what are you going to do about birth?" One husband replied by saying, "I will write a poem to welcome our baby."

Birthing is your time. It is your baby. It is your delivery. And I suggest you make your plans.

Remember as you write a birth plan, you have the right to change your mind at any time about any detail. Keep that in mind as you list your requests of how you would like things to be throughout labor. Birth plans are ways to open lines of communication among all members of your birthing team, and may include the following:

1. Ask your doctor for his routine hospital-admitting procedures. These procedures cover details about pubic shaving, enemas, use of an intravenous, and consumption of liquids.

2. Can you be up and about? When would any staff member insist that you go to bed? You may be comfortable lying down only during a portion of each hour. (When you lie down, position yourself on your side to take the weight of your uterus off large blood vessels in your pelvic cavity.)

3. Ask about showers. Can you take them? How long can you remain in there? Can your partner be with you?

4. Fetal monitoring. This was previously discussed, but what negotiation do you want to make on the subject?

5. Medications. Which drugs does your doctor normally use? When are they used? Discuss the use of medications and anesthetics in relationship to a cesarean section.

6. Take time to discuss the use of epidurals, spinals, or any other form of pain relief provided by your medical group.

7. Discuss the rupture of membranes and the consequence of labor not proceeding immediately thereafter.

8. At what point would your doctor rupture your membranes and what reason would he give to do so?

9. A discussion about the atmosphere in which you would prefer to labor and deliver. You may insist that a quiet, loving atmosphere is important to you.

10. Insist on the right to ask any staff members to leave the room if they are not being agreeable with your wishes. Remember, you are paying their salaries and providing the equipment they are working with on a daily basis. If you make no headway, request that the supervisor be present, or the department head, or the supervisor for the building. You never have to put up with surly behavior, a dripping tap, an overflowing diaper pail, or a lack of assistance with nursing your baby. Continue to request that your needs be met. The medical staff is available to meet your needs. If they fail to do this, then they will go out of business.

11. Talk with your doctor about the many issues of episiotomy.

12. Discuss the use of different positions for your baby's delivery: lying on your side, standing in an upright position, or squatting.

13. Make sure you can touch your baby's head, if you wish to, when your baby's head crowns (or is showing).

14. Would your doctor agree to your using acupuncture to bring on your labor if your membrane ruptured and you did not naturally come into labor?

15. Voice your preference for your baby to be placed on your tummy with skin-to-skin contact. Let your health team know you understand that if your baby requires resuscitation, your baby will be whisked to the warming incubator.

16. Request a delay in the installation of the antibiotic eye ointment until your bonding time has occurred.

17. Recall that cutting the cord is a separation event for your baby (such as the first time you stayed away from home overnight). So, whoever cuts the cord ought to do so with a great degree of thoughtfulness and recognition of the event's importance.

18. On the subject of cesarean section, make it clear who can be present, such as your back-up coach, and obtain this in writing.

After you and your doctor sign your birth plan, carry copies of it with you so that you have authority to ask anyone who is not cooperating to leave.

As you attend the childbirth classes, and as you read and talk, you will find other details that are important to you. So keep lists of questions and keep asking. Do not hesitate to personally contact the head of the nursery or the head of the post-partum unit if you feel that you have special desires or requests that may not be considered usual. Believe me, the hospital wants you as a patient.

The first birth plan I ever worked with was that of a young woman who completed a prepared childbirth class with me. She telephoned me and relayed the following information: "I am due in two weeks. I am not married to the father. We are strongly considering giving the baby up for adoption. I have herpes and I do not want a cesarean section!"

First, we discussed the imminent cesarean section. I suggested that she prepare for it. I felt comfortable proposing that we pray about the herpes, although I had never done such a thing before. So right there on the telephone, we prayed that her herpes would not be active. We drew up a birth plan over the telephone, detail by detail.

She felt so strongly that, no matter what happened, she owed her baby a peaceful delivery. She wrote out her requests and took them to her doctor, who agreed to everything except her partner being in the shower. When her partner agreed to wear swimming trunks, the latter was also okayed by the doctor.

I was privileged to be present at this peaceful, loving birth event. The mother's partner and a friend labored with her. I remember so vividly that as soon as her baby's head was delivered, the baby opened her eyes wide and looked at everyone, still with her body and shoulders inside the mother. The doctor, partner, and friend were so excited, they shouted with joy. This mother in delivery, with one leg in the air, motioned everyone to be quiet as she gently pushed her baby out. The doctor honored, with great dignity and patience, each of her requests. It was indeed a privilege to watch a formerly distraught young woman pull her resources together and receive the peaceful, natural delivery she asked for.

Birth plans have become so significant, entire books, such as *Your Baby, Your Way*,[48] have been written to support you in your birth experience.

By taking all the other steps in pre-birth bonding, you can minimize your surprises. Do not skip the preparation step, or think it merely perfunctory. This step requires more than compiling a shopping list.

Your birth plan is a declaration by you, in writing, of exactly what you want. It is a contract with yourself. It is a very important tool, because it will allow you to remove all birth preparation details from your head and to place them before you for review and evaluation. See if there is anything that you have overlooked, and notice whether you are clear in your thinking about giving birth.

The best thing that list-making does is to give you a chance to review your own thoughts, place them in logical order, and see whether they make sense, whether they are clear to others, and whether they will produce the outcome you desire.

Few expectant parents do this. I know list-makers who drive their spouses and family crazy if a vacation, or even an evening out, is being planned. These same people may go into the delivery room without having so much as put pencil to paper on the subject of birth. The doctor asks them if they want a spinal, and they say, "Spinal? Oh, well, whatever you think best, doctor." I mean, they have not even thought about it before. You may think that I am exaggerating, and that being unprepared is unusual, but I assure you it is not.

Prepare for this major event in your life. Take out a sheet of paper and begin to write. Write down whatever comes into your head. Put it down randomly. Do not worry about it making sense or following a proper sequence. Begin by placing your thoughts—all of your thoughts—on paper.

Talk to your partner, talk to your parents and friends, and talk to your doctor. Review educational material, come back to your lists, and write some more. Review your lists, then begin placing the information in a logical order to see if it makes sense, to see if there are any holes, and to see if the pattern fits for you.

Writing goals has another purpose. It is the most powerful form of affirmation there is. Visualization is wonderful. Writing reinforces the visualization. It is like placing your order with the universe.

Write your order now. Do not wait a moment longer. Take out a sheet of paper. Even as you finish reading this chapter, begin to make your lists. Review your lists periodically. You will make changes and additions. Your list becomes your working tool!

You will use these lists in practical ways in the weeks ahead of you. Your lists will become the basis of your birth plan with your doctor, with the medical facility, and even with your own family. Your birth plan is a mutual contract, drawn up by all parties involved in the birth. It is not an ultimatum from the mother-to-be to the rest of the world. A participating father-to-be has an equal voice in the birth plan details. Remember, this is your script, your movie. Commence writing. The stage has been set.

Remember another important detail. You do not have to do anything your doctor tells you to do, and your doctor can do nothing without your permission. So, do not give in to something that you do not want, that you do not believe in, simply because this is the way your doctor has always done it.

On the other hand, your list may produce a tendency to become too dogmatic about things. Be willing to remain flexible. If your doctor recommends something to you in the middle of birth, do not refuse to do it simply because it is not on your list! Your list and all of your preparations provide you with a point of reference, a plan, which may need to be fine-tuned as you progress through the stages of giving birth.

9

Materialization

One of the most challenging things in life, in fact for some people, the *most* challenging thing in life is to move from the conceptual to the physical plane, that is, to turn dreams into reality.

Most of us do very well at thinking about the way we want things to be and not so well in producing those results in our life. The fact is, if you can conceive of an idea, you can produce it. All it takes is action.

Step nine in pre-birth bonding, PUT YOUR PLAN INTO ACTION, is probably the most important step. This is where you put into practice what you have learned. This is where those who *talk* a good game are separated from those who *play* a good game. This is where the universe finds out who is truly sincere about acting on his or her ideas.

It is one thing to write something on a sheet of paper; it is quite another to see it through.

I am laying particular emphasis on this point because I want every woman to have the ideal birth. I know that no one, ultimately, can produce that outcome but you. The mother and the father of the new baby have to insist on having things the way they want them. The doctors cannot do it, the nurses cannot do it, all the books and classes cannot do it.

The beginning of step nine is to maintain communication with everyone involved with the birth of your child. First, be sure you continue to communicate with the baby; with yourself; with your partner; with your family, including any younger children in the family, and the expectant grandparents. Be sure communication with your doctor is direct and open. Visit the place where you are going to give birth. If you intend to use a birthing center, take a tour several weeks before the expected date of the baby's arrival. Choose the room you want to be in. Visualize yourself using that room. Talk to the staff. Have every question answered: Who may be present? Can you have your favorite picture on the wall to look at and concentrate on during the contractions? Choose musical tapes to play while giving birth.

Thirty days prior to your delivery date, have your birth plan signed by your doctor. Put everything in writing: the birth methods that will be used, the methods and procedures used in case of unexpected developments, the equipment that will be used, the medications that will be administered, the bonding time with the baby, and the people who will be permitted to be with you during labor and birth. All these details and more need to be provided by you, because you are in charge of how you want the birth of your baby to be.

Through self-education, you have already explored most of these questions. During visualization, you have pictured how you want it to be. In your preparation, you have committed everything to writing. Now, by putting your plan into action, you will see it all the way through.

Like a magician, you are going to materialize ideas, producing them in your reality. Have you found ideas, thoughts, and concepts in this book which you can use?

Have you started using your pre-birth bonding techniques? Have you and your partner established a sharing time together?

Have you started your visualization techniques? Are you talking to your baby every day? Have you begun your self-education process? Are you having open discussions with your partner?

Most parents' ideas about preparing for childbirth revolve around making a list of names for the baby. Maybe, with luck, they may think about taking a class or two. Even then, they often do not go home and do their homework, but wait until each class session to practice breathing and relaxation techniques.

Thinking and talking about things is good, but action is where the results are to be found. Action takes courage. It takes belief in your convictions. It takes the strength to assume total responsibility for the outcome of things. Verbalize your convictions by writing them down. Put this list by your mirror and read it each day out loud. Talk to yourself in the mirror about your convictions, so that you establish in your own being and in your own words what those convictions are.

Talk openly and honestly about how you want things to proceed during the delivery. Most of us are satisfied to listen to the doctor tell us how it is going to be. It takes even more strength when having things your way means disagreeing with your doctor. These days more and more doctors are listening to what the patient wants and are trying hard to accommodate them, while considering sound medical practices. Still, there are some doctors who will not listen to you, who wish to do the deliveries their way, and that is that. It is going to take courage either to change doctors or to look that kind of doctor in the eye and kindly say, "Thank you, doctor, and this is the way it is going to be."

Taking the step toward materialization in any facet of your life frequently involves both minor and major confrontations. Here is a way to take the sting out of confrontations. Take the word "but" out of your vocabulary. "But" disempowers people. Mainly it disempowers you.

Look at the following two sentences: "I know you always use restraining straps, doctor, but I do not want them." This statement is confrontational and disempowering to the speaker.

"I know you always use restraining straps, doctor, and I do not want them." This sentence contains two statements of truth with no confrontation. They are simply two statements of fact.

Try another imaginary dialogue. "Thank you for telling me about the fetal monitor, doctor, but I will not be using one." This statement is confrontational.

"Thank you for telling me about the fetal monitor, doctor, and I will not be using one." This sentence is simply a statement of fact. It puts you in charge.

Next, eliminate the word *can't* from your vocabulary. Substitute "I choose not to." For the truth is, you can do anything you choose to do. There is no such thing as "can't." When the doctor says, "We can't do that," remember, that the doctor is really saying, "I choose not to do that." Make sure the doctor understands that you know she is making a choice about that. Asking a doctor to alter her choice is a great deal easier than getting a doctor to do something she thinks she "can't" do.

What does all this have to do with step nine in pre-birth bonding? Materialization begins when you understand that you are the cause in your life, not the effect of someone else. If you have not already begun to set aside a few minutes each day to be with the baby, you can pretend it is because you just "can't" right now for lack of time, or you can tell the truth and acknowledge that you are not doing it because you do not choose to, at this time. There is a world of difference. "Can't" allows us to hide behind our lack of results. The words, "I choose not to" place things squarely on the line.

Dr. Sheila Kitzinger suggests that in dealing with the medical profession there is a great value in repetition, often called the "technique of the broken record." When you repeat yourself quietly but firmly, you cannot be driven off course. Dr. Kitzinger's suggestions on special skills with which to negotiate the kind of care you want are discussed in her chapter "Saying What You Want" in *Your Baby, Your Way*.[49]

Now that you have read this far, go back and make a list of all the things you have resolved to do in connection with the birth of your baby. Determine how many of those things you have done. See how many you have started. Do not mentally beat yourself up if your list looks pretty dismal in terms of results. Just notice that and move on. Just do the best you can. You can have it be the way you want it to be. All it takes is your active participation. Hundreds of thousands of people each year read self-help books and say, "That's a good idea." The difference between those who reap the benefits of that good idea and those who do not is what step nine is about.

Making your own decisions about things also makes you responsible. Doctors will tell you, for instance, that you can have it exactly the way you want it, if you are willing to sign a waiver of responsibility. You may often be intimidated into doing it the doctor's way because of this. The doctor may say, "Well, if you do not want the fetal monitor, okay, but I'm going to have to ask you to sign this statement stopping us from using it." What the doctor is telling you is that if anything goes wrong, he does not want to be responsible. Most of us would rather have the doctor responsible than have ourselves be responsible. So, we go ahead and have the fetal monitor anyway, in spite of the fact that we have read all about it, studied its results, know full well that we do not have a need for it, and really do not want to use it; we know millions of babies are born without a fetal monitor. But the doctor tries to scare us. I have had several mothers-to-be come to me and say, "Well, if the doctor feels that strongly about it, maybe I better have it."

The problem with being subservient to the doctor is that it presupposes that the doctor is always right and that the doctor knows best. The truth is, very often it has nothing to do with what the doctor knows and has everything to do with what the doctor fears. These days, doctors recommend every precaution and every procedure known because more have been sued in the past quarter century than, perhaps, in the entire preceding history of humankind. Doctors have become moving targets in a firing range where there is not much cover. The only cover the doctor can find these days is to make sure that every possible step is taken to avoid every possible complication. One cannot reasonably fault doctors for this. Their careers and personal welfare are on the line.

Another reason doctors and hospitals "do things" is because that is the way "it has always been done." One example of this is a mother who told me recently of her decision not to allow silver nitrate drops to be put in her baby's eyes immediately after birth. She was aware that the drops burn and cause the baby's eyes to swell. Silver nitrate is used to protect against damage to the eyes by a venereal disease. In most states it is required by law that this protection be given to all newborns, even if the pregnancy check-ups show no signs of venereal disease.

When this mother-to-be took a tour of the hospital where she was planning to have her baby, she casually mentioned to the nurses that she did not wish her child to be administered silver nitrate eye drops. The nurse became defensive. "Oh, you have to," she told the expectant mother. "It's a state law."

Actually, the law gives parents the option of *either*

silver nitrate eye drops or an antibiotic ointment called erythromycin. This particular mother-to-be happened to know this. When she mentioned it, the nurse stiffened, "Well, it's the policy of the hospital to administer the silver nitrate eye drops."

What does a mother do in a case like this? She says simply, "I understand that is the policy of the hospital, and what is true is that silver nitrate is not required by law. Therefore, my baby will not have the eye drops, and I prefer the use of the antibiotic eye ointment."

The doctor and the hospital now are faced with a decision. Either they grant the wishes of the patient (the consumer) or they lose her business. You can insist on having it your way or you can choose another hospital or another doctor. The truth is, hospitals and doctors are in a service profession and neither care to lose patients. One hospital made a new policy concerning the use of silver nitrate because so many parents asked for the erythromycin. Silver nitrate eye drops were abandoned in favor of the eye ointment.

"Hospitals know women make the most health care decisions for their families," says Mary Anne Grof, president of the consulting firm, Health Care Innovations. So services geared to women serve as a gateway for future business to hospitals today.

Doctors control hospital purse strings by admitting patients, thereby running up the revenue. Hospitals are closing in the United States because they fail to respond to consumer needs, and because of the huge rise of outpatient services and short stays in hospitals, reported *U.S. News and World Report*, April 11, 1988. Realize that you are the source of income for the hospitals of the future.

Too often, the doctor and the hospital are in partnership, and the parents-to-be are bystanders with no decision-making powers at all. The point is not to place yourself in an adversarial relationship with your doctor and hospital, but to place yourself in a partnership. This is what I mean by choosing to be the cause rather than the effect. You are not caught up in the effect of someone else's decisions or policies, unless, of course, you agree with them.

Step nine of pre-birth bonding involves more than doctors, nurses, and hospitals. It includes everybody who will play a role in the birth of your child.

I recall one story of a young mother-to-be who wanted her husband at her side during the delivery. "But I guess I just can't," she sighed. When I inquired why this was so, she rolled her eyes to heaven and said, "My mother won't allow it. She says she doesn't care what anybody says, that's no place for a man. I can't talk her out of it."

The grandmother-to-be may have believed that if the husband were there, her own role in the birth would be diminished. I suggested that the young woman let her mother know, once more, what her wishes were— not as a request, but as a simple explanation of how the birth was going to be.

Still another mother was reluctant to have her baby in an Alternative Birthing Center, even though, from what she had read about them, she felt she wanted to very much. She explained that her birthing instructor did not think it was a very good idea, notwithstanding the fact that birthing centers have been operating successfully for years.

Birthing centers, unlike most hospital rooms, look very much like your bedroom at home. The labor and delivery takes place in the same room, in a normal bed, rather than on a thin metal slab of a table, minus all the hospital paraphernalia. There are drapes on the windows, carpets on the floor, rockers and easy chairs for family members, to be with the mother and observe the birth if they wish. There are pictures on the walls, even a tape deck to play your favorite music. This mother start had read about Alternate Birthing Centers in a number of books and knew that this was where she wanted to have her baby. However, her pre-birth class instructor had, for reasons not clear, some prejudice against birthing centers. By the time the eight-week class was completed, the mother-to-be, again thinking that the instructor must know best, reluctantly decided to have the baby in a more clinical setting after all.

This illustrates what I mean when I say that step nine, put your plan into action, is the most important step in the whole scheme—and it takes the most courage. One of my recommendations here is to read an array of books about the childbirth process (see the Suggested Reading list). As you acquire information from additional sources, such as tapes, lectures, and classes, decide for yourself exactly how you want the birth to be. Then, set out to make it happen that way.

10

Actualization

Step ten, EXPERIENCE THE BIRTH, is the actual event of having your baby—utilizing your education and all you have visualized and materialized, and bringing it into your experience. You may think experiencing the birth is not a step at all in pre-birth bonding since it seems like the end result of all the other steps, but it can also be labeled as "follow through." As such, it is most definitely a step on its own.

Here you are, at the eleventh hour. The time has come for the new life that you and your partner have created and nurtured to come into the outer world. This is the time you have been waiting for. The most important thing I can say of this time is, forget everything else you have ever heard, read, been told, learned, or decided about what it is like to have a baby.

The most important three words I would ever say to a mother at the hour of the birth of her child is to "be here now." Some of the decisions made prior to this moment will be thrown out the window, and that is perfectly all right. The birthing room is no place to be dogmatic. It is a place to trust what you know intuitively to be perfect for the moment.

I remember a mother who had taken many weeks of classes to learn the proper way to breathe during a natural delivery. When the time came she found that she did not want to do what she was taught. It seemed to be going okay with her just breathing naturally, normally, without using any specific technique. Then her husband, who was with her in the delivery room, began urging her to breathe the way she was taught in class.

"I don't want to!" she said.

"Come on, honey!" her husband sincerely urged. "This is the way we are supposed to do it, remember?"

So she dutifully started her breathing routine and promptly hyperventilated. Before they could help her calm down, she fainted.

Another mother, in the midst of her labor, just "had a feeling that something was wrong." Earlier, she had said rather firmly that she did not want a fetal monitor during labor, but something told her to stay with her experience, which was one of inexplicable uneasiness. She called the nurse and ordered the monitor.

"But your chart says no monitor," the nurse replied.

"Thank you, nurse. I know what I decided earlier, and I've changed my mind."

This is a case of a woman who knew that, in the end, nothing mattered except "the way it is now." As it happened, there was no complication, but the state of relaxation that her decision produced in her made the delivery go more smoothly than it might have had she become more and more distraught while ignoring some silent inner-warning signal.

You will enjoy the birth of your baby as you have never enjoyed anything before if you will follow this simple rule: "Set aside all your pictures." *Pictures* is a term I use to mean preconceived notions of how the birth can be. As I said before, this may seem to be a contradiction of all that I have written earlier. Actually it is not. I have said, you can have the birth of your

baby be exactly the way you want it, and that is true.
What I have not stated, until now, is that *how* you want
it to be may change, as your intuitive knowledge
changes right there on the spot.

It is important to maintain complete freedom of
choice right up to, and including, the very moment your
baby is born.

What you decide in these moments may not fit into
your mind's earlier pictures of how the birth was going
to be. Do not let that defeat you.

In the majority of cases, things will go as planned
with only minor deviations. But these deviations sometimes can be annoying to expectant parents who have
everything established in their mind's eye and can brook
no interference with these pictures. Such a posture may
make things unnecessarily difficult for you.

There is another reason to let go of your pictures
and "be here now," at the moment of your baby's birth.
There is magic in the moment if you live it as it happens, rather than through the veil of your expectations.
When you are in the here and now, you make decisions
more rapidly and with more clarity. Your senses are
heightened. Your wisdom comes to the fore, and your
choices are almost automatic. It has passed the time
when you and I can be wishy-washy about how we give
birth to our children. How many babies will you have
in your family? Families of eleven children are not so
common today. Each birthing experience is one of
importance for every family member. All details of birth
are important and can be pursued with great vigor.
Every time you and I make a move toward natural
birth, it is a step toward a world returned to its natural
purpose.

One couple, LeAnn and Steve Jamison, pursued
every detail about their second birth. Their story is one
of a mother empowering herself and her baby, examining at length the possibilities of materializing and

actualizing her personal desires for birth. In LeAnn's own words:

In our first labor, like most people, we wanted a natural delivery and we believed we had a doctor who supported that philosophy. During the delivery, I had no control. The control was taken away from me. There were no choices, and it was all decided for me by the medical profession.

My membranes ruptured early one morning, and I was admitted to the hospital. I was put to bed, given an intravenous with the drug Pitocin to induce labor, but my body did not respond. Neither was I allowed to get out of bed. After some twelve hours of hard labor, I had only dilated one centimeter. So I was given an epidural and more Pitocin. My internal feeling was that this is not natural. They are trying to tear my baby away from me. Three hours after the epidural was given, my cervix was fully dilated. Pushing was also difficult, for my baby was not coming out.

My memory of this stage of labor is of the anesthesiologist literally doing pushups on the upper end of my uterus, my husband curling my shoulders up and also pushing me. The obstetrician was using suction cups two or three times to deliver the baby, finally resorting to the use of metal forceps. In my mind, I couldn't believe it. They were tearing this baby out of me.

For my second delivery, I sought an obstetrician, Dr. David Priver, who I felt confident was absolutely invested in natural childbirth and doing whatever that means.

About three weeks prior to my second delivery, I was told by the examining nurse that my baby was in a breech presentation. The nurse duly went through all the implications of hospital admission, turning the baby, or doing a breech vaginal delivery.

Remembering my first delivery and the difficulty with the delivery of my baby's head, I was not anxious to do a breech vaginal delivery. I was reassured that no obstetrician would force me to do that, and it was suggested to me that I talk to the baby about turning down. I consulted with psychologist David Chamberlain over the telephone. My husband whispered low over my abdomen and talked to our baby about turning. I sent strong mental images to my baby.

Three days later, on a Monday morning, I was examined at my doctor's office, and my baby was found to be a head presentation. So, I was all set now for delivery. I talked with my husband about our birth plan and all significant details of who was to be present when we gave birth.

I ruptured my membranes first, exactly the same commencement to labor as with my first baby. I stayed home, went into the shower, and used nipple stimulation and love play to encourage the onset of contractions and labor.

Later in the day, I was admitted to a labor, delivery, and recovery room in a hospital. I used no drugs, no monitoring, other than a (monitoring) strip to prove that all was well with the baby. I remained up and about and I felt in total control of birth. My baby and I worked together for a healthy delivery. My baby was born in a posterior position, that is, with the baby's face uppermost, which causes the baby's back to be against my spine. My baby did not cry when she was born but was calm and at total peace. I never anticipated so much pleasure from birth.

My gratitude to my obstetrician is enormous. I thank him for his guidance, support, and being there for me. My doctor was tuned into my needs and made helpful suggestions such as, 'A lot of ladies like a hot shower when their cervix is almost fully dilated.' My doctor suggested moving from my being on all fours when pushing the baby out, into a squatting position, to see if it would be more comfortable for me.

My delivery, my birthing, was an experience that left all three of us at peace with the world.

LeAnn believed that you can and do have the ability to manifest your wishes; you and your baby may enjoy a positive birth process. Psychologist Arthur Janov validates LeAnn's experience; he writes in his book *Imprints*:[50]

The nine months of development and growth in the mother's womb can alter and even damage many physiological processes, especially in those precious hours before birth, the feeling, remembering, and experiencing fetus may battle for or against coming into life. This may cause traumas during and around birth that are permanently engraved as imprints on the fragile, developing nervous system of the newborn. Those birth imprints shape later personality and physiotype, determine physiological and neurological responses and direct the very behavior pattern we eventually manifest. That same imprint assists to determine whether we will be constant travelers, compulsive workers, heavy smokers, alcoholics, asthmatics, epileptics, aggressive or passive beings.

🌰

One can describe events that occur during the pregnancy, labor and delivery, and early life as being laid down like a cellular "thumbprint" which we carry for life. Quite often, the imprints are obvious if we listen to what we say. Dr. Janov refers to them as "primal slips."

I had experienced this in my own life long before I read Janov's work. Once in the middle of a marital spat with my husband, I said, "You did not want me in the first place anyway." My husband and I both stopped in our conversational tracks. We realized simultaneously that the statement was directed at my mother and not at him. The truth is that I was a child born of a wealthy, single woman, in an age when that was an embarrassment. Needless to explain, I had run all my relationships around the fact of not being wanted. Always believing that at some point I would be rejected, I had always been ready for flight.

These conversational slips often occur when you ask a friend, "How are you doing?" Notice the use of the statements: "I am stuck." "I am under pressure." "I am being pulled in all directions." These are three examples of thirty or more primal slips listed in Dr. Janov's book.

The power of thought and imprinting around birth is illustrated by a personal experience of Paul Brenner, an obstetrician well-known for his metaphysical presentations relating to birth and death. In his book, *Life is a Shared Creation*,[51] he tells about studying as a medical student for his national boards. During this laborious process, he prayed that if he ever did have a child, the child would never, ever have to study in panic as he had done most of his life. He added very strongly that he wanted his child to be a musician, a person who could share with others his life's work, and a person whose hobby would be his life's work. Dr. Brenner had a son who, when he grew up, went through college, and then, to everyone's surprise, became a rock guitarist.

Recently on television, I viewed a powerful program on teenage suicide. One of the parents made a passionate statement: While she was pregnant, she wished her child had died. This wish was so heavily imprinted by her frequent repetition throughout the pregnancy that she felt it was left in the child's mind. At sixteen years of age, the child killed himself.

Other imprints can be nutritional. While speaking at a college on the subject of imprinting, I reminded the class that there was a period of time in the United States when the majority of obstetricians suggested to women that they gain no more than ten pounds during pregnancy. Many pregnant mothers attempted to please their doctors by doing this. Immediately one young woman in the class shot her hand up to tell us how her mother did exactly that. She had been starved, she told us. Then, she detailed to us what her mother's diet was at the time.

This was a class studying child development, but out of curiosity, I asked the student, "Is food important to you?" "Yes," the young woman replied, "it absolutely runs my life. I never stop thinking about it. In fact, guess what I'm graduating from college in?" Her college major was culinary arts.

If a pregnant mother chooses to keep her blood sugar shooting up and down by drinking soda pop all day, it is not surprising that her child will crave and react to sugar later on. Stress, a high intake of fat, and starvation have profound chemical effects on the unborn child, through adrenalin being released. As Dr. Janov points out, chemical imprints are lifelong.

The actualization of birth is also affected by the time period in which we live. For us, technology has a significant impact.

As we look back in history, we find a true story about Dr. Ignaz Philipp Semmelweis, chronicled in the historical novel, *The Cry and the Covenant*.[52] In part, it tells how hand-washing was introduced into obstetrics just over a century ago. The custom of the time dictated that when people died, their bodies were cut up and examined by doctors. The more blood you had on your coat, the better doctor you were. After doing postmortems, the doctors wiped their hands on their coats and went on immediately to do deliveries. The women of Europe cried in the streets, for they did not want to be admitted into hospitals where they knew they might die. So, Dr. Semmelweis made a change. He put a bowl of water (later, an antiseptic solution) at the entrance of the maternity wards, and required all of his medical students to wash their hands.

Anthropologist Robbie Davis-Floyd has analyzed the relationship between women and doctors in the age of technology. Often, it has been implied that men are superior to women and women's bodies are regarded as defective machines. Dr. Davis-Floyd says that the core values of society are reflected in birth, and by our rituals around birth. "Why would we need to learn about our cultural habits?" she asks. One answer is, women are the primary socializers of our children, and if women are conveying, through our current births, that everything is mechanical, birth is technological, women's bodies are inferior, men are superior, and surgical intervention is best, then that is what our children will learn.

Dr. Davis-Floyd examines technological birth and suggests that technological assistance may be valuable and useful, but you may be overpowered by the control desired by others. She suggests that you do not lay down your autonomy when you lie down during the birthing process. She asks you to look at your value system, society's value system, the rituals and systems of birth in your section of society. This will help you to make some distinct choices about what you want. The rituals and implications of technology and the potential interference are many, from the use of a wheelchair for being admitted, to the separation of husband and wife, to the use of an intravenous (which looks like a symbolic placental cord), to lying down on one's back to give birth.

As you prepare for birth and observe modern hospital rituals, always remember that the ritual can be changed; you have the power to bring about the change.

I have been impressed by some couples whose

jaundiced babies had to remain in the hospital nursery for one or two days under phototherapy lights. (Before fluorescent lights were discovered to break down the extra red blood cells that cause the yellow pigmentation, jaundiced babies were subjected to risky blood exchange transfusions.) They set up routines so that one parent was always present in the nursery with the newborn. This is an example of modern technology combined with the loving care of parents.

Frequently, a baby is returned to the hospital's nursery at night so the mother can rest. If you abide by this ritual, and you are breast-feeding, you can insist that your baby be brought out to you during the night, as needed. Also, give the nursery staff written instructions not to give your baby a bottle of formula during the night.

Abandoning the practice of sending healthy newborns to nurseries is being suggested because studies show that babies do much better when they stay with their mothers. In South America, a study was done on premature babies who normally would have been kept in an incubator. Instead, they were bound to the warmth of their mother's chest. Hearing the mother's heartbeat, being stimulated by the mother's breathing, and having milk on demand, these babies had a higher rate of survival than similar babies kept in incubators.

In the light of technology, let us browse through *The Birth of a Father*,[53] Martin Greenberg's personal experiences during the birth of his child. In it, he writes about the immediate use of a wheelchair—hospital policy, of course—which implies that pregnant women are not able to walk, even though walking during early labor is an excellent thing to do. Dr. Greenberg talks about the nurse asserting her authority by retrieving a stethoscope from him, the father, and depriving him of the pleasure of listening to his baby's heartbeat, and perhaps, saying to his baby, "All is well. You are handling labor beautifully." He describes the bleak, white, stark labor room, then the implied defectiveness of the mother's body, as the medical staff becomes impatient because she is not proceeding quickly enough in labor. So, the decision is made to "break the waters." Scheduling and production within a given time frame seem to take priority in our modern technological world.

As the membranes are ruptured, an internal monitor (a fine wire screwed into the baby's scalp) is put into use. Labor now becomes intense. Dr. Greenberg writes, "The machine had taken her over. It [the monitor] was physically located where I had been sitting." Here is a medical person scared to touch the monitor because after all, another doctor had placed it where he wanted it. Sometimes we, the medical profession, manage to fill very small labor rooms with a great deal of medical equipment. Dr. Greenberg was not able to wipe his wife's brow or whisper words of encouragement. Finally, he moves the machine and the bed. He squeezes in beside his wife. Now, he is able to watch the monitor and observe the contractions, but he is very aware that he is annoying the staff. He feels proud to help his wife, and his wife lets him know that he is assisting her well.

When the contractions become very strong, and his wife is wondering if she can take it anymore, her doctor visits and lets her know she is doing fine. The nurse, however, shakes her head and say loud enough for all to hear, "This woman is not going to push the baby out." The doctor attempts to salvage the situation, but Dr. Greenberg feels lost in a sea of negativism with no support. The labor progresses to the pushing phase and everyone ends up in the delivery room.

The description of the episiotomy is unpleasant as he watches their doctor snip away at his wife. Because of the time factors of modern obstetrics and because the mother is lying on her back for delivery, the forceps are used to pull the baby out. His wife gives one final huge push. The baby is delivered, and the joy and the power of birth takes over in the delight of the new baby.

Joseph Chilton Pearce, author of *Magical Child*,[54] in his chapter, "Breaking the Bond," is critical of hospital birth. He talks about how medical interference and the use of drugs are stresses on the baby and may lead to loss of muscle coordination and synchronization. His description of how the staff grabbed the baby's fantastically fragile head are heart-wrenching. Following these ghastly descriptions of birth he depicts the isolation of the baby in the nursery.

Pearce points to differences between our technologically born babies' sleeping habits and those of the Ugandan naturally born babies. Researcher Marcelle Geber found that the babies she studied in Uganda slept less and were more alert than American babies. When supported by the forearms at only forty-eight hours after birth, these Ugandan babies had head balance, eye focus, and showed marvelous alertness. The babies who had been studied crawled at six or seven weeks, which is not found in American babies until six months. Pearce, in his scathing words about us abandoning our babies to nurseries, asks, "What is being built into the very fibers of the mind/brain/body system as the initial experiences of life?" He observes, our babies are experiencing unrelenting stress in their first encounters with people. Frequently, the initial contact with the world is through material objects.

Pearce's observations in his book have serious implications of personal responsibility for those of us choosing modern hospital deliveries. In the event your baby has to go to an intensive care unit, arrange to stay with your baby. Have the lighting reduced, artificially create night and day; get rid of the rock music overhead, and insist that the noise levels be reduced. Make use of Dr. Ruth Rice's infant massage,[55] talk lovingly and reassuringly to your baby, and watch your baby respond and recover more quickly than those not receiving such personal attention.

A baby brings consciousness and intelligence with him from the time he develops in the mother's womb and his heart begins to beat. Just as we actually bond with and love our child long before he is born, we can take that extra step immediately after the baby's birth.

I have devoted a great portion of my life to ensure wonderful births for babies all over the world, from Australia to England to America. My concern has grown in recent years as my understanding of the information which babies are learning from the beginning of life grows. I can think of nothing more important to do than to improve our birth experiences. The tomorrows of this world depend on what we do with the todays. The people who will populate those tomorrows will make their own choices, but we, as parents, influence them from the time they are in the womb.

Your child begins his education the moment he gains consciousness in the womb, not at the moment of birth. Love your child from the moment you learn there is to be a child. Love him in all your thoughts, all your words, all your actions. Love your baby from the very beginning. This, more than anything will produce the happy ending you desire.

CREATION

They talk about creative genius,
Of artists, authors, scientists and statesmen;
But you and I together, beloved,
A man and a woman, average in talent,
Possess the precious power to create,
Through our ennobling love for one another,
An actual human being, a baby,
Who then will grow, mature, become an adult,
And full-fledged member of the human race,
With infinite potentialities,
For happiness, achievement, service to man.
This gift sublime of creativity,
Bestowed by Nature on all living things,
Expands, enriches love's essential meaning,
Makes everyone in love a kind of god,
And blesses human sexuality,
As the wonderful and happy way,
To guarantee a future for mankind.

—Corliss Lamont, *"Lover's Credo"*[56]

Pre-Birth Bonding Steps

1. *REST*—Set aside time, at least ten minutes, each day for mother and father to be together, to rest and just to be with the baby. Establishing such a daily routine can benefit the family relationship long after the baby is born.

2. *ENJOY THE BABY*—In step one you are just being there with the baby. After about a week or so, begin to actively talk about the baby. Talk about the coming months, your plans, your hopes, your dreams.

3. *MAKE CONTACT WITH THE BABY*—Send thoughts to your baby. No matter what stage of pregnancy you are in, communicate your growing awareness of the baby and your love for him/her. Enhance the time you set aside to spend with the baby by playing music you enjoy. Send relaxing, loving thoughts to the baby as you rest a hand on mother's stomach. The baby will be able to experience your touch and your love.

4. *BEGIN CONVERSATION*—When you are ready, add voice to thought, music, and touch. Put your thoughts into words, adding a new dimension to the relationship between mother, father and baby.

These are the first building blocks to a three-way communication.

5. *SHARE YOUR WHOLE LIFE*—Increase the amount of time you spend with your unborn child. Include your baby in every aspect of your life. Communicate with your baby at all times, using thoughts and words. Establish a link which involves the lives of mother, father, baby, and any other family members.

6. *VISUALIZE*—Set aside a time each day to use the power of visualization to begin planning exactly how the birth of your child will be. Use your mind as a chalkboard to draw specific images.

7. *EDUCATE YOURSELF*—Attend classes and lectures; read books, magazine, and newspaper articles; view videotapes and television programs; talk to doctors, nurses, midwives and other new mothers. Leave no question unanswered as you begin to make basic decisions about the birth of your child.

8. *PREPARE FOR THE BIRTH*—Make lists of all your ideas and birth plans. Be specific. Try to think of everything, then think it through again. Discuss your plans and thoughts with your partner and baby. Prepare a written agreement—a birth plan—and have your doctor sign it thirty days prior to your due date. Communicate clearly with every person to be involved with the birth process. Continue to rest, think and talk to the baby, touch the baby, and play music.

9. *PUT YOUR PLAN INTO ACTION—* Materialize your plans. Tour the location where you plan to give birth. Check every detail, such as who will stand in if your doctor is unavailable when the baby comes. Continue your education, exploring your thoughts, using visualizations in preparation for birth.

10. *EXPERIENCE THE BIRTH*—Enjoy the birth event. Forget everything you have read or heard about birthing a baby. Throw out all old "pictures." Trust your intuition to tell you what to do as the event unfolds. This is the most rewarding experience you, your partner, and your baby will ever share.

Appendix

SUGGESTED VIDEOS

A Gift for the Unborn Child. 1985. Bradley Boatman Productions, Malibu, CA. Distributed by Ferde Grofe Films, Inc., 4091 Glencoe Avenue, Marina Del Rey, CA 90292, (213) 827-1168.

Active Birth. Balaskas, Janet. Video on Life Productions. Available from ICEA Bookcenter (listed below).

Baby Basics. 1987. Vida Health Communications, Inc. Available from ICEA Bookcenter (listed below).

Knowing the Unborn. 1988. Ballard, Royda, with Kelley Ballard. Distributed by Pre-Birth Parenting, 2554 Lincoln Blvd., Ste. 509, Marina Del Rey, CA 90291, (213) 417-3663.

Journey to be Born: An Introduction to Pre- and Perinatal Psychology. 1986. Findeisen, Barbara. STAR Foundation, 3960 W. Sausal Lane, Healdsburg, CA 95448, (707) 857-3475.

The Miracle of Life. 1983. Nilsson, Lennart. Boston: WGBH Educational Foundation. (Shown on the PBS broadcast series, "Nova.") Available from ICEA Bookcenter (listed below).

Prepare and Celebrate Pre- and Postnatal Exercise Programs for Life. 1987. Jain, Katherine DaSilva. 5 Mt. Tioga Ct., San Rafael, CA 94903, (415) 492-9497. Also available from ICEA Bookcenter (listed below).

Tender Touch: A Guide to Infant Massage. 1987. Healthy Alternatives, Inc. Available from ICEA Bookcenter (listed below).

Your Baby Is Worth the Weight. James, Pam, and Lilly Meehan. (Prenatal nutrition.) 125 Eliot St., Santa Paula, CA 93060, (805) 525-1882.

SUGGESTED MUSIC

Aura, William. "Timeless" and "Miracles." 1982. Available at most music stores. William Aura Music, 1775 Old Country Rd., Ste. 8, Belmont, CA 94002.

Bartels, Joan. "Lullaby Magic." Discovery Music, 4130 Greenbush Ave., Sherman Oaks, CA 91423, (800) 451-5175.

Bearns, Robert, and Ron Dexter. 1977. "Golden Voyage." Awakening Productions Inc., 4132 Tuller Ave., Culver City, CA 90230.

Halpern, Steve. A tape series available at most music stores. Halpern Sounds. 1775 Old Country Road., Ste. 9, Belmont, CA 94002.

Jones, Alex, and Doug Cutler. 1982. "Kali's Dream: Peaceful Piano Melodies." P.O. Box 161, Claremont, Ontario, LOH IEO Canada.

Kelly, Georgia. A tape series available at most music stores. Heru Records, P.O. Box 954, Topanga, CA 90290.

Murooka, Hajime. 1974. "Lullaby From the Womb." Toshiba. E.M.I. 845 Via de la Paz, Ste. 454, Pacific Palisades, CA 90272.

Thurman, Leon, and Anna Peter Langness. "Heartsongs." Music Study Services, Englewood, CO 80155.

Verny, Thomas, M.D., and Sandra Collier. "Love Chords." A & Records of Canada, Scarborough, Ontario.

Vivaldi, Antonio. "Four Seasons." Various recordings, available at most music stores.

Vollenweider, Andreas. 1986. "Behind the Gardens— Behind the Wall—Under the Moon" and "Down to the Moon." CBS Records. Available at most music stores.

SUGGESTED READING

Arms, Suzanne. 1975. *Immaculate Deception*. New York: Bantam Books.

Baldwin, Rahima. 1979. *Special Delivery; The Complete Guide To Informed Birth*. Berkeley, CA: Celestial Arts.

Barr, Linda, and Catherine Monserrat. 1979. *Teenage Pregnancy: A New Beginning*. Buena Park, CA: Morning Glory.

Brewer, Gail Sforza, ed. 1978. *The Pregnancy After 30 Workbook*. Emmaus, PA: Rodale Press, Inc.

Brewer, Gail Sforza, with Tom Brewer, M.D. 1985. *What Every Pregnant Woman Should Know: The Truth About Diet and Drugs in Pregnancy*. New York: Penguin Books.

Brewer, Sforza Gail. 1988. *The Very Important Pregnancy Program: A Personal Approach to the Art and Science of Having a Baby*. Emmaus, PA: Rodale Press, Inc.

Chamberlain, David. 1988. *Babies Remember Birth*. Los Angeles: Jeremy P. Tarcher, Inc.

Cohen, Nancy Wainer, and Lois J. Estner. 1983. *Silent Knife: Cesarean Prevention and Vaginal Birth After Cesarean*. South Hadley, MA: Bergin and Garvey Publishers, Inc.

Dick-Read, Grantly, M.D. 5th edition, 1984. *Childbirth Without Fear*. New York: Perennial Library, Harper and Row.

Edwards, M. 1984. *Reclaiming Birth*. 1984. Trumansburg, NY: The Crossing Press.

Elkins, Valmai Howe. 1985. *The Rights of the Pregnant Parent*. New York: Schocken Books.

English, Jane. 1985. *A Different Doorway: Adventures of a Cesarean Born*. Point Reyes Station, CA: Earth Heart.

Ewy, Donna, and Rodger Ewy. 1984. *Teen Pregnancy*. Boulder, CO: Pruett Publishing.

Gaskin, Ina May. 1978. *Spiritual Midwifery*. Summertown, TN: Book Publishing Co.

Gaskin, Ina May. 1987. *Babies, Breastfeeding and Bonding*. Granby, MA: Bergin & Garvey Publishers, Inc.

Gawain, Shakti. 1978. *Creative Visualization*. Mill Valley, CA: Whatever Publishing.

Gold, E.J. and C. Gold. 1977. *Joyous Childbirth: A Manual For Conscious Child Birth*. Berkeley, CA: And/Or Press.

Greenberg, Martin. 1985. *The Birth of a Father*. New York: Continuum.

Heinowitz, Jack. 1982. *Pregnant Fathers*. Englewood Cliffs, NJ: Prentice Hall.

ICEA members, and Doris Haire. "The Pregnant Patient's Bill of Rights," and "The Pregnant Patient's Responsibilities." Available from ICEA Bookcenter (listed below). (800) 624-4934.

Inch, Sally. 1984. *Birthrights*. New York: Pantheon Books.

Kitzinger, Sheila. 1980. *The Complete Book of Pregnancy and Childbirth.* New York: Penguin.

Klaus, Marshall, M.D., and Phyllis Klaus. 1985. *The Amazing Newborn.* Reading, MA: Addison-Wesley Publishing Co., Inc.

Leach, Penelope. 1982. *Your Baby and Child.* New York: Knopf.

McCutcheon-Rosegg, Susan, and Peter Rosegg. 1984. *Natural Childbirth, the Bradley Way®.* New York: Dutton.

Nilsson, Lennart. 1976 rev. ed. *A Child Is Born: The Drama of Life Before Birth.* New York: Delacorte Press.

Noble, Elizabeth. 1983. *Childbirth with Insight.* 1983. Boston, MA: Houghton Mifflin Co.

Ohashi, Wataru, with Mary Hoover. 1983. *Natural Childbirth, The Eastern Way.* New York: Ballantine Books.

Olkin, Sylvia K. 1987. *Positive Pregnancy Fitness: A Guide to a More Comfortable Pregnancy and Easier Birth Through Exercise and Relaxation.* Wayne, NJ: Avery.

Peterson, Gayle H. 1981. *Birthing Normally: A Personal Growth Approach To Childbirth.* Berkeley, CA: Mindbody Press.

Peterson, Gayle H., and Lewis Mehl. 1985. *Cesarean Birth-Risk and Culture.* Berkeley, CA: Mindbody Press.

Richards, Lynn Baptisti, et al. 1987. *The Vaginal Birth After Cesarean (VBAC) Experience.* South Hadley, MA: Bergin and Garvey Publishers, Inc.

Rothman, Barbara Katz. 1982. *In Labor: Women and Power in the Birth Place.* New York: Norton.

Shapiro, Jerrold L. 1987. *When Men Are Pregnant: Needs and Concerns of Expectant Fathers*. San Luis Obispo, CA: Impact Pubs Cal.

Simkin, Penny, Janet Whalley, and Ann Keppler. 1984. *Pregnancy, Childbirth, and the Newborn*. Deephaven, MN: Meadowbrook Books.

Stukane, Eileen. 1985. *The Dream Worlds of Pregnancy*. New York: Quill.

OTHER INFORMATION SOURCES

ASPO/Lamaze. American Society for Psychoprophylaxis in Obstetrics. (Parents are welcome as members.) 1840 Wilson Blvd., Ste. 204, Arlington, VA 22201, (703) 524-7802.

Birth and Life Bookstore. 7001 Alonza Ave. N.W., P.O. Box 70625, Seattle, WA 98107, (206) 789-4444. Over 1,200 titles on childbirth, child care, breast-feeding, and related subjects. Write for free copy of newsletter, "Imprints," which includes reviews and an annotated booklist.

ICEA (International Childbirth Education Association) Bookcenter. P.O. Box 20048, Minneapolis, Minnesota 55420, (612) 854-8660 or (800) 624-4934. ICEA Bookcenter's catalog, "Bookmarks," includes an annotated list of books on childbirth, family-centered maternity care, breast-feeding, and early child care.

National Organization of Circumcision Information Resource Center. P.O. Box 2515, San Anselmo, CA 94960, (415) 488-9883.

Bibliographic References

CHAPTER ONE

1. Chamberlain, David B., M.D. 1988. *Babies Remember Birth*. Los Angeles: Jeremy P. Tarcher, Inc.

   see also:

   Chamberlain, David B., M.D. 1987. "The Cognitive Newborn: A Scientific Update." *British Journal of Psychotherapy*. Vol. 4 (1): 30-71.

CHAPTER THREE

2. Janov, Arthur. 1983. *Imprints: The Lifelong Effects of the Birth Experience*. New York: Coward-McCann.

   Janov, Arthur. 1980. *The Primal Scream*. New York: G.P. Putnam's Sons, Perigee Books.

3. Rossi, Ernest L., and David B. Cheek, M.D. 1988. *Mind-Body Therapy: Methods of Ideodynamic Healing in Hypnosis*. New York: W.W. Norton.

4. Pearce, Joseph C. 1980. *Magical Child: Rediscovering Nature's Plan for Our Children*. New York: Bantam Books.

5. Greenberg, Martin, M.D. 1985. *The Birth of a Father*. New York: Continuum.

6. Heinowitz, Jack, M.D. 1982. *Pregnant Fathers*. Englewood Cliffs, NJ: Prentice Hall.

CHAPTER FOUR

7. Peale, Norman Vincent. 1956. *The Power of Positive Thinking*. New York: Fawcett Crest Books.

8. Peale, Norman Vincent. 1982. *Positive Imaging*. New York: Fawcett Crest Books.

9. Holmes, Ernest, and Willis Kinnear. 1959. *A New Design for Living*. Los Angeles: Science of Mind Publications.

10. Pearsall, Paul. 1986. *Superimmunity*. New York: McGraw-Hill.

11. Siegel, Bernie S., M.D. 1986. *Love, Medicine and Miracles*. New York: Harper & Row, Publishers, Inc.

12. Hay, Louise L. 1984. *You Can Heal Your Life*. Santa Monica, CA: Hay House, Inc.

13. Rice, Ruth D., M.D. 1978. *The Loving Touch Book*. Dallas, TX: Cradle Care, Inc.

14. Montagu, Ashley. 1971. *Touching*. New York: Harper & Row Publishers, Inc.

   see also:

   Montagu, Ashley. 1965. *Life Before Birth*. New York: New American Library.

15. Ludington-Hoe, Susan, with Susan Golant. 1987. *How To Have a Smarter Baby*. New York: Bantam Books.

16. Nilsson, Lennart. 1976 rev. ed. *A Child Is Born*. New York: Delacorte Press.

17. Lumley, Judith M., M.D. 1982. "Attitudes to the Fetus Among Primigravidae." *Australian Paediatric Journal*. 18:106-109.

18. Nilsson, Lennart. *The Miracle of Life*. 1983. Boston: WGBH Educational Foundation. (Part of the PBS series, "Nova." Video also available through ICEA Bookcenter.)

CHAPTER FIVE

19. Vollenweider, Andreas. "Behind the Gardens—Behind the Wall—Under the Tree." Also, "Down to the Moon." CBS Records. Available at most music stores.

20. McKenna, James. 1986. "An Anthropological Perspective on the Sudden Death Syndrome." *Medical Anthropology Quarterly.*

21. DeCasper, Anthony. 1987. "Human Fetuses Eavesdrop in the Womb: Data and Implications." Paper presented at the 3rd International Congress on Pre- and Perinatal Psychology, San Francisco, CA.

    DeCasper, Anthony, and M. Spence. 1982. "Prenatal Maternal Speech Influences Human Newborn's Auditory Preferences." Paper presented at the 3rd Biennial International Conference on Infant Studies, Austin, TX.

    DeCasper, Anthony, and M. Spence. 1986. "Prenatal Maternal Speech Influences Human Newborn's Auditory Perception of Speech Sounds." *Infant Behavior Development.* 9:133-50.

22. Verny, Thomas, M.D., with John Kelly. 1981. *The Secret Life of the Unborn Child.* New York: Dell Publishing.

23. Thurman, Leon, and Anna Peter Langness. "Heartsongs." Music Study Services, Englewood, CO.

24. Verny, Thomas, M.D., and Sandra Collier. "Love Chords." A & Records: Scarborough, Ontario, Canada.

25. Laibow, Rima E., M.D. 1986. "Birth Recall: A Clinical Report." *Pre- and Perinatal Psychology Journal.* 1:1, 78-81.

26. Freeman, Marc. 1987. "Is Infant Learning Egocentric or Duocentric? Was Piaget Wrong?" *Pre- and Perinatal Psychology Journal*. 2:1, 25-42.

27. Odent, Michel, M.D. 1984. *Entering the World*. New York: Marion Boyars Publishers, Inc.

28. Mehl, Lewis, E., M.D. 1981. *Mind and Matter*. Berkeley, CA: Mindbody Press.

CHAPTER SIX

29. Davis-Floyd, Robbie. 1986. "Birth as an American Rite of Passage." University Microfilms Publication No. 86-18448 (dissertation abstracts). Department of Anthropology/Folklore, University of Texas, Austin, TX.

30. McKay, Susan. 1986. *The Assertive Approach to Childbirth*. Minneapolis, MN: International Childbirth.

31. Peterson, Gayle H. 1981. *Birthing Normally: A Personal Growth Approach to Childbirth*. Berkeley, CA: Mindbody Press.

see also:

Peterson, Gayle H. 1987. "Prenatal Bonding, Prenatal Communication and the Prevention of Prematurity." *Pre- and Perinatal Journal of Pyschology*. 2:2, 87-92.

32. Star, Rima B. 1986. *The Healing Power of Birth*. Austin, TX: Star Publishing.

see also:

Star, Rima B., and Steven Star. 1982. *Celebration, The Underwater Birth of Mela Noel*. Austin, TX: Star Publishing.

33. Maybruck, Patricia, M.D. 1986. "An Exploratory Study of Pregnant Women's Dreams." University Microfilms International. University of Michigan, Ann Arbor, Michigan.

Maybruck, Patricia, M.D. 1989. *Dreams and the Pregnant Mind*. Los Angeles: Jeremy P. Tarcher, Inc. (*Note: not released at LoveStart publication date; 1989 expected release date*)

34. Kitzinger, Sheila. 1987. *Your Baby, Your Way*. New York: Pantheon Books, Inc.

CHAPTER SEVEN

35. Notzon, Francis C., Paul J. Placek, and Selma M. Taffel. 1987. "Comparisons of National Cesarean-Section Rates." *The New England Journal of Medicine*. 316:7, 386-89.

36. Caldeyro-Barcia, Roberto, M.D. 1979. "The Influence of Maternal Position on Time of Spontaneous Rupture of the Membranes, Progress of Labor, and Fetal Head Compression." *Birth and the Family Journal*. 6:1, 7-15.

37. Gaskin, Ina May. 1978. *Spiritual Midwifery*. Summertown, TN: Book Publishing Co.

Gaskin, Ina May. 1987. *Babies, Breastfeeding and Bonding*. Granby, MA: Bergin & Garvey Publishers, Inc.

38. Banta, H. David, M.D., and Stephen B. Thacker, M.D. 1979. "Electronic Fetal Monitoring: Is It of Benefit?" *Birth and the Family Journal*. 6:4, 237-249.

39. Thacker, Stephen B., M.D. 1987. "The Efficacy of Intrapartum Electronic Fetal Monitoring." *American Journal of Obstetrics and Gynecology*. 156:1, 24-30.

40. Caldeyro-Barcia, Roberto, M.D. 1979. "The Influence of Maternal Position." *Birth and the Family Journal.* 6:1, 7-15.

   See also:

   Caldeyro-Barcia, Roberto, M.D., *Birth and the Family Journal* reprints available through ICEA Bookcenter, e.g., "Some Consequences of Obstetrical Interference," and "The Influence of Maternal Bearing-down Efforts During the Second Stage on Fetal Well-Being."

41. Anand, K.J.S., M.D., and P.R. Hicky, M.D. November 19, 1987. "Pain and Its Effects in the Human Neonate and Fetus." *The New England Journal of Medicine.*

42. ICEA. 1988. "Epidural Anesthesia for Labor." *International Journal of Childbirth Education.* 3:1, 24 (special supplement).

43. Odent, Michel, M.D. 1984. *Birth Reborn.* New York: Pantheon Books, Inc.

44. Kitzinger, Sheila. 1986. *Being Born.* New York: Grossett and Dunlap.

45. Kitzinger, Sheila. 1987. *Your Baby, Your Way.* New York: Pantheon Books.

46. Thacker, Stephen B., M.D., and David H. Banta, M.D. 1983. "Benefits and Risks of Episiotomy: An Interpretive Review of the English Language Literature 1860-1980." *Obstetrical and Gynecological Survey.* 38:6, 322-334.

CHAPTER EIGHT

47. Montagu, Ashley. 1971. *Touching.* New York: Harper & Row Publishers, Inc.

48. Kitzinger, Sheila. 1987. *Your Baby, Your Way*. New York: Pantheon Books, Inc.

CHAPTER NINE

49. Kitzinger, Sheila. 1987. *Your Baby, Your Way*. New York: Pantheon Books.

CHAPTER TEN

50. Janov, Arthur. 1983. *Imprints: The Lifelong Effects of the Birth Experience*. New York: Coward-McCann.

51. Brenner, Paul. 1981. *Life Is a Shared Creation*. Marina Del Rey, CA: DeVorss and Co.

52. Thompson, Morton. 1951. *The Cry and the Covenant*. London: William Heinemann Ltd.

53. Greenberg, Martin, M.D. 1985. *The Birth of a Father*. New York: Continuum.

54. Pearce, Joseph C. 1980. *Magical Child: Rediscovering Nature's Plan for Our Children*. New York: Bantam Books.

55. Rice, Ruth D., M.D. 1978. *The Loving Touch Book*. Dallas, TX: Cradle Care, Inc.

56. Lamont, Corliss. 1972. "Creation," in *Lover's Credo*. New York: A.S. Barnes and Company.

If you would like to receive a catalog of products and information about future workshops, lectures and events sponsored by the Louise L. Hay Educational Institute which assists people in loving themselves, please detach and mail the postcard below.

I would like to be placed on the Hay House, Inc. mailing list.

NAME＿＿＿＿＿＿＿＿＿＿＿＿＿＿＿＿＿＿＿＿

ADDRESS＿＿＿＿＿＿＿＿＿＿＿＿＿＿＿＿＿＿

＿＿＿＿＿＿＿＿＿＿＿＿＿＿＿＿＿＿＿＿＿

Book in which this card was attached:

＿＿＿＿＿＿＿＿＿＿＿＿＿＿＿＿＿＿＿＿＿

HAY HOUSE, INC.
P. O. Box 2212
Santa Monica, CA 90406